Genetic Screening and Counseling

Guest Editors

ANTHONY R. GREGG, MD
JOE LEIGH SIMPSON, MD

OBSTETRICS AND GYNECOLOGY CLINICS OF NORTH AMERICA

www.obgyn.theclinics.com

Consulting Editor
WILLIAM F. RAYBURN, MD, MBA

March 2010 • Volume 37 • Number 1

SAUNDERS an imprint of ELSEVIER, Inc.

W.B. SAUNDERS COMPANY

A Division of Elsevier Inc.

Elsevier, Inc. ● 1600 John F. Kennedy Blvd. ● Suite 1800 ● Philadelphia, PA 19103-2899

http://www.theclinics.com

OBSTETRICS AND GYNECOLOGY CLINICS OF NORTH AMERICA Volume 37, Number 1
March 2010 ISSN 0889-8545, ISBN-13: 978-1-4377-1843-0

Editor: Carla Holloway

Obstetrics and Gynecology Clinics (ISSN 0889-8545) is published quarterly by Elsevier Inc., 360 Park Avenue South, New York, NY 10010-1710. Months of issue are March, June, September, and December. Periodicals postage paid at New York, NY, and additional mailing offices. Subscription price per year is $257.00 (US individuals), $431.00 (US institutions), $130.00 (US students), $309.00 (Canadian individuals), $544.00 (Canadian institutions), $191.00 (Canadian students), $376.00 (foreign individuals), $544.00 (foreign institutions), and $191.00 (foreign students). To receive student/resident rate, orders must be accompanied by name of affiliated institution, date of term, and the signature of program/residency coordinator on institution letterhead. Orders will be billed at individual rate until proof of status is received. Foreign air speed delivery is included in all *Clinics* subscription prices. All prices are subject to change without notice. POSTMASTER: Send address changes to *Obstetrics and Gynecology Clinics*, Elsevier Health Sciences Division, Subscription Customer Service, 3251 Riverport Lane, Maryland Heights, MO 63043. **Customer Service: Telephone: 1-800-654-2452 (U.S. and Canada); 314-447-8871(outside U.S. and Canada). Fax: 314-447-8029. E-mail: journals customerservice-usa@elsevier.com (for print support); journalsonlinesupport-usa@elsevier.com (for online support).**

Reprints. For copies of 100 or more of articles in this publication, please contact the Commercial Reprints Department, Elsevier Inc., 360 Park Avenue South, New York, New York 10010-1710. Tel.: 212-633-3818; Fax: 212-462-1935; E-mail: reprints@elsevier.com.

Obstetrics and Gynecology Clinics of North America is also published in Spanish by McGraw-Hill Interamericana Editores S.A., P.O. Box 5-237, 06500, Mexico; in Portuguese by Reichmann and Affonso Editores, Rio de Janeiro, Brazil; and in Greek by Paschalidis Medical Publications, Athens, Greece.

Obstetrics and Gynecology Clinics of North America is covered in MEDLINE/PubMed (Index Medicus), Excerpta Medica, Current Concepts/Clinical Medicine, Science Citation Index, BIOSIS, CINAHL, and ISI/BIOMED.

Printed and bound by CPI Group (UK) Ltd, Croydon, CR0 4YY

Transferred to Digital Print 2011

GOAL STATEMENT

The goal of *Obstetrics and Gynecology Clinics of North America* is to keep practicing physicians up to date with current clinical practice in OB/GYN by providing timely articles reviewing the state of the art in patient care.

ACCREDITATION

The *Obstetrics and Gynecology Clinics of North America* is planned and implemented in accordance with the Essential Areas and Policies of the Accreditation Council for Continuing Medical Education (ACCME) through the joint sponsorship of the University of Virginia School of Medicine and Elsevier. The University of Virginia School of Medicine is accredited by the ACCME to provide continuing medical education for physicians.

The University of Virginia School of Medicine designates this educational activity for a maximum of 15 *AMA PRA Category 1 Credits*™ for each issue, 60 credits per year. Physicians should only claim credit commensurate with the extent of their participation in the activity.

The American Medical Association has determined that physicians not licensed in the US who participate in this CME activity are eligible for a maximum of 15 *AMA PRA Category 1 Credits*™ for each issue, 60 credits per year.

Category 1 credit can be earned by reading the text material, taking the CME examination online at http://www.theclinics.com/home/cme, and completing the evaluation. After taking the test, you will be required to review any and all incorrect answers. Following completion of the test and evaluation, your credit will be awarded and you may print your certificate.

FACULTY DISCLOSURE/CONFLICT OF INTEREST

The University of Virginia School of Medicine, as an ACCME accredited provider, endorses and strives to comply with the Accreditation Council for Continuing Medical Education (ACCME) Standards of Commercial Support, Commonwealth of Virginia statutes, University of Virginia policies and procedures, and associated federal and private regulations and guidelines on the need for disclosure and monitoring of proprietary and financial interests that may affect the scientific integrity and balance of content delivered in continuing medical education activities under our auspices.

The University of Virginia School of Medicine requires that all CME activities accredited through this institution be developed independently and be scientifically rigorous, balanced and objective in the presentation/discussion of its content, theories and practices.

All authors/editors participating in an accredited CME activity are expected to disclose to the readers relevant financial relationships with commercial entities occurring within the past 12 months (such as grants or research support, employee, consultant, stock holder, member of speakers bureau, etc.). The University of Virginia School of Medicine will employ appropriate mechanisms to resolve potential conflicts of interest to maintain the standards of fair and balanced education to the reader. Questions about specific strategies can be directed to the Office of Continuing Medical Education, University of Virginia School of Medicine, Charlottesville, Virginia.

The faculty and staff of the University of Virginia Office of Continuing Medical Education have no financial affiliations to disclose.

The authors/editors listed below have identified no professional or financial affiliations for themselves or their spouse/partner: Jeffrey S. Dungan, MD; Janice G. Edwards, MS, CGC; Gary Fruhman, MD; Nancy S. Green, MD; Susan Hiraki, MS; Carla Holloway (Acquisitions Editor); William Irvin, MD (Test Author); Susan Klugman, MD; Krista B. Moyer, MGC; Thomas W. Prior, PhD; and Ignatia B. Van den Veyver, MD.

The authors/editors listed below identified the following professional or financial affiliations for themselves or their spouse/partner:
Anthony R. Gregg, MD (Guest Editor) is on the Advisory Committee/Board for Novartis Diagnostics.
Susan J. Gross, MD is an industry funded research/investigator for PerkinElmer Inc., is an industry funded research/investigator and consultant for Luminex Molecular Diagnostics Inc., has an educational grant from Genzyme, and has a patent pending with Einstein Medical School.
Thomas J. Musci, MD is a consultant for DNA Direct, and is employed by Novartis Diagnostics.
William F. Rayburn, MD, MBA (Consulting Editor) is an industry funded research/investigator and a consultant for Cytokine PharmaSciences.
Lee P. Shulman, MD is an industry funded research/investigator for Bayer; is on the Advisory Committee/Board for Bayer, Ortho, and Schering-Plough; and is employed by GSK, Sanofi Pasteur, Merck, Bayer, Ortho, and Schering-Plough.
Joe Leigh Simpson, MD (Guest Editor) is on the Advisory Committee/Board for Bayer Healthcare and Biox Dx, and owns stock in Biocept.
Peggy Walker, MS owns stock in Genzyme Corp and 3M.

Disclosure of Discussion of non-FDA approved uses for pharmaceutical products and/or medical devices:

The University of Virginia School of Medicine, as an ACCME provider, requires that all faculty presenters identify and disclose any off-label uses for pharmaceutical and medical device products. The University of Virginia School of Medicine recommends that each physician fully review all the available data on new products or procedures prior to clinical use.

TO ENROLL

To enroll in the Obstetrics and Gynecology Clinics of North America Continuing Medical Education program, call customer service at 1-800-654-2452 or visit us online at www.theclinics.com/home/cme. The CME program is available to subscribers for an additional fee of $195.00

Contributors

CONSULTING EDITOR

WILLIAM F. RAYBURN, MD, MBA
Randolph Seligman Professor and Chair, Department of Obstetrics and Gynecology;
Chief of Staff, University Hospital, University of New Mexico Health Science Center,
Albuquerque, New Mexico

GUEST EDITORS

ANTHONY R. GREGG, MD
Associate Professor, Director, Division of Maternal Fetal Medicine, Medical Director,
Clinical Genetics and Molecular Medicine, Department of Obstetrics and Gynecology,
University of South Carolina School of Medicine, Columbia, South Carolina

JOE LEIGH SIMPSON, MD
Executive Associate Dean for Academic Affairs; Professor of Human and Molecular
Genetics; Professor of Obstetrics and Gynecology, College of Medicine, Florida
International University, Miami, Florida

AUTHORS

JEFFREY S. DUNGAN, MD
Associate Professor, Division of Clinical Genetics, Department of Obstetrics and
Gynecology, Northwestern University Feinberg School of Medicine, Chicago, Illinois

JANICE G. EDWARDS, MS, CGC
Clinical Professor and Director, Genetic Counseling Program, University of South Carolina
School of Medicine, Columbia, South Carolina

GARY FRUHMAN, MD
Genetics Resident, Department of Molecular and Human Genetics, Baylor College
of Medicine, Houston, Texas

NANCY S. GREEN, MD
Associate Professor, Department of Pediatrics, Columbia University Medical Center,
New York, New York

ANTHONY R. GREGG, MD
Associate Professor, Director, Division of Maternal Fetal Medicine, Medical Director,
Clinical Genetics and Molecular Medicine, Department of Obstetrics and Gynecology,
University of South Carolina School of Medicine, Columbia, South Carolina

SUSAN J. GROSS, MD
Professor, Obstetrics and Gynecology and Women's Health, Albert Einstein College
of Medicine; Chair, Obstetrics and Gynecology, North Bronx Health Care Network,
Bronx, New York

SUSAN HIRAKI, MS
MPH Candidate, Mailman School of Public Health, Columbia University, New York, New York

SUSAN KLUGMAN, MD
Associate Professor, Obstetrics and Gynecology and Women's Health, Albert Einstein College of Medicine; Director, Reproductive Genetics, Montefiore Medical Center, Bronx, New York

KRISTA MOYER, MGC
San Francisco Perinatal Associates, Inc; Clinical Laboratories, University of California San Francisco Medical Center, San Francisco, California

THOMAS J. MUSCI, MD
San Francisco Perinatal Associates, Inc, San Francisco, California

THOMAS W. PRIOR, PhD
Professor, Director of Molecular Pathology, Department of Pathology, The Ohio State University, Columbus, Ohio

LEE P. SHULMAN, MD
The Anna Ross Lapham Professor in Obstetrics and Gynecology, Chief, Division of Clinical Genetics; Co-Director, Northwestern Ovarian Cancer Early Detection and Prevention Program; Department of Obstetrics and Gynecology; Director, Cancer Genetics Program; Robert H. Lurie Comprehensive Cancer Program, Feinberg School of Medicine of Northwestern University; Adjunct Professor of Medicinal Chemistry and Pharmacognosy; University of Illinois at Chicago College of Pharmacy, Chicago, Illinois

IGNATIA B. VAN DEN VEYVER, MD
Associate Professor, Departments of Obstetrics and Gynecology and Molecular and Human Genetics, Baylor College of Medicine, Houston, Texas

PEGGY WALKER, MS
Genetic Counselor, Division of Clinical Genetics and Molecular Medicine, Clinical Assistant Professor, Department of Obstetrics and Gynecology, University of South Carolina School of Medicine, Columbia, South Carolina

Contents

(AJ) descent are at increased risk of having offspring with particular genetic diseases that have significant morbidity and mortality. In addition, there are some disorders, such as cystic fibrosis, for which northern European Caucasians are at comparable risk with those of an AJ background. Carrier screening for many of these Jewish genetic disorders has become standard of care. As technology advances, so does the number of disorders for which screening is available. Thus, we need to continue to be cognizant of informed consent, test sensitivity, confidentiality, prenatal diagnosis, preimplantation genetic screening, and public health concerns regarding testing.

Cystic fibrosis is the first genetic disorder for which universal screening of preconceptional or prenatal patients became a component of standard prenatal care. The molecular genetics and mutation profile of the CFTR gene are complex, with a wide range of phenotypic consequences. Carrier screening can facilitate risk assessment for prospective parents to have an affected offspring, although there remains a small residual risk for carrying a mutation even with a negative screening result. There are ethnic differences with respect to disease incidence and effectiveness of carrier testing, which may complicate counseling.

Healthy women who carry a "premutation" in the FMR1 gene (or fragile X mental retardation protein) can pass on a further mutated copy of FMR1 to either male or female offspring, leading to fragile X syndrome (FXS). Premutation carriers do not have manifestations of FXS in cognitive deficits, behavioral abnormalities, or classic physical features, but are at increased risk for development of the "fragile X–associated disorders": premature ovarian insufficiency and fragile X–associated tremor and ataxia syndrome. When considering widespread prenatal carrier screening programs for fragile X, significant resources must be available for at-risk individuals, including counseling, accurate diagnostic options for fetal testing, and choice regarding continuation of a pregnancy. Further attention is needed to develop and utilize inexpensive screening tests with adequate sensitivity and specificity to reduce barriers to screening for the population. Recently newer methodologies for high-throughput and inexpensive screening assays, which correctly detect expanded alleles in premutation and full mutation patients with a high degree of sensitivity, show significant promise for reduction in cost with rapid turn around times. With the introduction of widespread screening, individuals will be made aware not only of their risk for offspring with FXS, but will also have knowledge of the potential risk to develop the adult-onset conditions- FXPOI and FXTAS. This introduces more complex counseling challenges. All individuals identified as carriers of intermediate or premutation alleles should be referred for genetic counseling to properly convey risks for allele expansion and to discuss possible future risks of fragile X–associated disease.

Applications of Array Comparative Genomic Hybridization in Obstetrics

Gary Fruhman and Ignatia B. Van den Veyver

Current prenatal cytogenetic diagnosis uses mostly G-banded karyotyping of fetal cells from chorionic villi or amniotic fluid cultures, which readily detects any aneuploidy and larger structural genomic rearrangements that are more than 4 to 5 megabases in size. Fluorescence in situ hybridization (FISH) is also used for rapid detection of the common aneuploidies seen in liveborns. If there is prior knowledge that increases risk for a specific deletion or duplication syndrome, FISH with a probe specific for the region in question is done. Over the past decade, array-based comparative genomic hybridization (aCGH) has been developed, which can survey the entire genome for submicroscopic microdeletions and microduplications, in addition to all unbalanced chromosomal abnormalities that are also detected by karyotype. aCGH in essence interrogates the genome with thousands of probes fixed on a slide in a single assay, and has already revolutionized cytogenetic diagnosis in the pediatric population. aCGH is being used increasingly for prenatal diagnosis where it is also beginning to make a significant impact. The authors review here principles of aCGH, its benefits for prenatal diagnosis and associated challenges, primarily the inability to detect balanced chromosomal abnormalities and a small risk for discovery of chromosomal abnormalities of uncertain clinical significance. The superior diagnostic power of aCGH far outweighs these concerns. Furthermore, such issues can be addressed during pre- and posttest counseling, and their impact will further diminish as the technology continues to develop and experience with its prenatal diagnostic use grows.

Screening, Testing, or Personalized Medicine: Where Do Inherited Thrombophilias Fit Best?

Peggy Walker and Anthony R. Gregg

Inherited thrombophilias present an opportunity to review population-based screening paradigms. Inherited thrombophilias are a group of complex conditions, and women who carry mutations in implicated genes have an increased risk of adverse pregnancy outcomes as well as venous thromboembolism. That asymptomatic carriers are at risk of manifesting phenotypes moves these conditions out of the traditional molecular genetic "screening" paradigm. Like most complex disorders, residual risk remains after molecular testing for thrombophilia, and the magnitude of this risk has not been quantified. Family and personal history are important factors to consider when providing personal risk assessment to patients. Overall, "testing" for thrombophilias according to a personalized medicine model is more appropriate than population "screening" as performed in other mendelian genetic conditions.

Hereditary Breast and Ovarian Cancer (HBOC): Clinical Features and Counseling for BRCA1 and BRCA2, Lynch Syndrome, Cowden Syndrome, and Li-Fraumeni Syndrome

Lee P. Shulman

This article provides an overview of the molecular changes associated with inherited gynecologic malignancies and the incorporation of this information in the counseling of individuals at increased risk for developing malignancies, as well as conventional and emerging approaches to the screening of the general population. Cancer genetic counseling and its role in women's health care is examined. The focus is hereditary breast and ovarian cancer; however, cancer predisposition caused by genes other than *BRCA1* and *BRCA2* is also considered. The aim is to provide a foundation for counseling based on fundamental knowledge of the genes and their clinical consequences. The reader is then guided through the mechanics of risk assessment for individual patients, concluding with the psychosocial implications of counseling.

FORTHCOMING ISSUES

June 2010
Update on Medical Disorders in Pregnancy
Judith Hibbard, MD, *Guest Editor*

September 2010
**Management of Complications from
Gynecologic Surgery**
Howard Sharp, MD, *Guest Editor*

December 2010
Cosmetic Procedures in Gynecology
Doug Laube, MD, *Guest Editor*

RECENT ISSUES

December 2009
Challenging Issues in Women's Health Care
Kathleen Kennedy, MD, *Guest Editor*

September 2009
**Female Pelvic Medicine and Reconstructive
Surgery**
Joseph I. Schaffer, MD, *Guest Editor*

June 2009
Women and Obesity
Raul Artal, MD, *Guest Editor*

RELATED INTEREST

Surgical Clinics of North America August 2008 (Vol. 88, Issue 4)
Hereditary Cancer Syndromes
Ismail Jatoi, MD, PhD, FACS, *Guest Editor*
www.surgical.theclinics.com

THE CLINICS ARE NOW AVAILABLE ONLINE!

Access your subscription at:
www.theclinics.com

Foreword

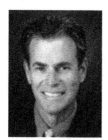

William F. Rayburn, MD, MBA
Consulting Editor

This issue, edited by Anthony Gregg, MD, and Joe Leigh Simpson, MD, is a much needed update of the 2002 issue pertaining to genetic screening and counseling for obstetrician-gynecologists. The purpose of this issue is to assist obstetrician-gynecologists in understanding and applying the concepts of molecular genetics to clinical practice, research, and the provision of health care in the community. In conjunction with genetics counselors, this issue reviews the basics of contemporary prenatal counseling. This issue of *Obstetrics and Gynecology Clinics* on genetics contains all of the current topics of active clinical relevance.

Human genetics and molecular testing are playing an increasing role in obstetric and gynecologic practice. As the practice of medicine evolves, so too does screening for potentially treatable genetics conditions. It is essential that obstetrician-gynecologists be aware of the advances in understanding of genetic disease and the fundamental principles of evolving technologies, molecular testing, and genetic screening.

As described in this issue, the "genomics era" of gene identification, characterization of disease-causing mutations, and advances in genetic technology have led to an increased number of available tests for the diagnosis of genetic disorders (eg, cystic fibrosis, fragile X syndrome, spinal muscular atrophy, inherited thrombophilias, and disorders in Ashkenazi Jews), carrier detection, and prenatal or preimplantation genetic diagnosis. Testing for a specific genetic disorder often occurs in an obstetric setting based on family history, a couple's ethnicity, or a past fetal condition.

In addition to prenatal diagnoses, this issue focuses on counseling for hereditary breast and ovarian cancer. An estimated 5% to 7% of all breast and ovarian cancer is attributed to inherited mutations in two highly penetrant, autosomal dominant susceptibility genes, *BRCA1* and *BRCA2*. *BRCA* testing in the presence of multiple family members affected with breast or ovarian cancer or a family in which a BRCA mutation has been discovered can reduce anxiety if negative or to explore various management options if positive.

All disorders currently considered for population screening are reviewed here and all by authoritative authors. Readers should find these articles readily applicable for

Obstet Gynecol Clin N Am 37 (2010) xiii–xiv
doi:10.1016/j.ogc.2010.04.002
0889-8545/10/$ – see front matter © 2010 Elsevier Inc. All rights reserved.

their practices. In the future, elucidation of the genetic basis for more reproductive disorders, common diseases, and cancer with improved technology for genetic testing will expand testing opportunities and influence prevention strategies and treatment options.

William F. Rayburn, MD, MBA
Department of Obstetrics and Gynecology
University of New Mexico School of Medicine
MSC10 5580, 1 University of New Mexico
Albuquerque, NM 87131-0001, USA

E-mail address:
wrayburn@salud.unm.edu

Preface:

Genetic Screening and Counseling

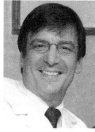 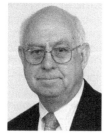

Anthony R. Gregg, MD   Joe Leigh Simpson, MD
Guest Editors

When the first edition of *Genetic Screening and Counseling* was published in 2002,[1] the draft of the human genome had just been declared sequenced.[2] Since then, the sequence has become nearly finalized, and the focus is turning to translation of this information to the bedside. The genomics era is increasingly bearing fruit and promises a paradigm shift in research and medical practice. To the clinician, counseling and genetic diagnoses will become an increasing part of daily practice. The generalist obstetrician/gynecologist is included.

Our first edition was prompted by successful joint efforts of the American College of Obstetricians and Gynecologists (ACOG), The American College of Medical Genetics (ACMG), and the National Institutes of Health (NIH). Guidelines were established for cystic fibrosis carrier screening, the first panethnic genetic disorder recommended for population screening solely through molecular (DNA) approaches. This agreement was soon followed by recommendations from professional societies to assimilate and incorporate additional genetics knowledge into daily practice. But there are obvious impediments, not just physicians increasing their genetic awareness, but finding a method to communicate to our patients. How can this be accomplished in the context of a busy practice? To help explain how, we have teamed in this edition with genetics counselors who provide their perspective. We have also expanded our scope to include an article on newborn screening, given increasing attention by ACOG, ACMG, March of Dimes, American Academy of Pediatrics, and Health Education Resources Services Administration. All these organizations state that successful implementation of newborn screening starts with an informed obstetrician.

All disorders currently considered for population screening are reviewed here, and all by authoritative authors. Thomas Prior covers carrier screening for spinal muscular atrophy. Thomas Musci and Krista Moyer consider the merits and technical and

Obstet Gynecol Clin N Am 37 (2010) xv–xvi
doi:10.1016/j.ogc.2010.04.001
0889-8545/10/$ – see front matter © 2010 Elsevier Inc. All rights reserved.

counseling controversies surrounding screening for fragile X syndrome. Screening for conditions common among the Ashkenazi Jewish population is covered by Susan Klugman and Susan Gross, who specifically recommend expanded screening in this ethnic group. Jeffrey Dungan addresses nuances in the ACOG/ACMG recommendations for cystic fibrosis carrier screening.

Our scope also extends beyond prenatal screening and counseling per se, targeting two areas in which significant progress has been made. Genetic screening and counseling for thrombophilias are discussed, illustrating well the concept of personalized medicine. Genetic counseling and screening for cancers—now pivotal to women's health—are discussed by Lee Shulman. Finally, to illustrate the technology driving us in new directions, array CGH (comparative genomic hybridization) is discussed by Ignatia Van den Veyver and Gary Fruhman. This diagnostic method is already used in research and clinical oncology, and could complement if not replace traditional karyotyping in prenatal diagnosis.

We believe you will find these articles readily applicable for your practice. Genetic screening and counseling are indeed an integral part of obstetrics and gynecology.

Anthony R. Gregg, MD
Division of Maternal Fetal Medicine
Clinical Genetics and Molecular Medicine
Department of Obstetrics and Gynecology
University of South Carolina School of Medicine
Two Medical Park, Suite 208
Columbia, SC 29203, USA

Joe Leigh Simpson, MD
Department of Obstetrics and Gynecology
College of Medicine
Florida International University
11200 SW 8th Street, HLS 693
Miami, FL 33199, USA

E-mail addresses:
Anthony.Gregg@uscmed.sc.edu (A.R. Gregg)
simpsonj@fiu.edu (J.L. Simpson)

REFERENCES

1. Gregg AR, Simpson JL, editors. Genetic screening and counseling. Obstet Gynecol Clin North Am 2002;29(2):255–396.
2. Lander ES, Linton LM, Birren B, et al. Initial sequencing and analysis of the human genome. Nature 2001;409:860–921.

Contemporary Genetic Counseling

Janice G. Edwards, MS, CGC

KEYWORDS

- Genetic counseling • Genetic services
- Obstetrician gynecologist • Resources

Providing care for women thoughout their life is a privilege and a responsibility. Obstetrician gynecologists have the opportunity to forge trusting connections with women in their reproductive years through middle age and beyond. These physician advisors hear women's concerns and provide medical insights into health care decisions that are often unique for female patients. The role of genetics in health and illness creates a large responsibility for physicians including recognizing genetic risk and exploring appropriate interventions with patients. Clinicians must continually realign their knowledge to incorporate the growing role of genetics in medicine. This article considers the contemporary use of genetic counseling for the obstetrician gynecologist, and how genetic counselors can serve as a resource to the physician and the patient.

CONNECTING WITH GENETIC COUNSELING RESOURCES

Genetic professionals are available in most academic medical centers and larger hospital systems. Genetic counselors serve as an educational resource for physicians and their staff, and provide genetic evaluation and counseling for referred individuals and their families. Genetic counseling services span the life cycle from preconception counseling to infertility evaluation, prenatal genetic screening and diagnosis, and include predisposition evaluation and genetic diagnosis for a growing number of adult onset conditions. Genetic professionals include American Board of Medical Genetics (ABMG) certified clinical geneticists (MD) and laboratorians certified in their genetic subspecialties of molecular genetics, cytogenetics and/or biochemical genetics (PhD).[1] The American Board of Genetic Counseling (ABGC) certifies Master of Science–prepared genetic counselors who typically provide direct care to patients and their families, sometimes with a geneticist and as an independent care provider.[2]

Genetic Counseling Program, University of South Carolina School of Medicine, Two Medical Park, Columbia, SC 29203, USA
E-mail address: jedwards@uscmed.sc.edu

Obstet Gynecol Clin N Am 37 (2010) 1–9
doi:10.1016/j.ogc.2010.01.003   obgyn.theclinics.com

The National Society of Genetic Counselors (NSGC) recently redefined genetic counseling in this contemporary perspective[3]:

Genetic counseling is the process of helping people understand and adapt to the medical, psychological, and familial implications of genetic contributions to disease. This process integrates the following:

- Interpretation of family and medical histories to assess the chance of disease occurrence or recurrence
- Education about inheritance, testing, management, prevention, resources, and research
- Counseling to promote informed choices and adaptation to the risk or condition.

Genetic counselors have traditionally worked in concert with obstetricians in reproductive medicine and with pediatricians in the evaluation of children with genetic conditions and birth defects. Adult-focused genetic counseling has grown exponentially as our understanding of single gene and complex conditions has evolved. For instance, since the identification of cancer susceptibility genes, BRCA1/2, genetic counselors routinely interact with surgeons, oncologists, and other cancer specialists managing risk for inherited predisposition. As our understanding of complex genetic disease continues to unfold, genetic counselors will increasingly offer input into other medical specialties, most recently in the area of cardiology. Genetic counselors serve physicians and their patients at all stages of the life cycle, and are expected to increase their role in subspecialty care as the use of genetic information becomes further integrated into medicine.

Laboratory-based genetic counselors are a unique consultative resource for physicians. Genetic testing takes place in a myriad of settings including academic genetic laboratories, national reference laboratories, and specialized molecular genetics laboratories. As a physician seeks current information about testing options, laboratory genetic counselors are available to counsel the clinician about ordering appropriate genetic testing and assist in interpretation of results, including referral to local genetic counseling services. Obstetricians are encouraged to connect with the genetic counselor liaison associated with most genetic laboratories for assistance in coordinating appropriate genetic testing.

Genetic counselors practice in all 50 states, and can be located through medical schools or hospitals in addition to genetic laboratories, typically in larger cities. The NSGC estimates more than 2600 genetic counselors currently practice in the United States, and more than 200 enter the profession annually, graduating from 1 of 32 ABGC accredited training programs.[4] The profession is growing in the United States with several new training programs under development. Internationally, there are now Master of Science genetic counselor education programs in 16 countries spanning 5 continents, with several countries considering how to create the profession to strengthen their genetic service delivery systems.[5]

The NSGC Web site maintains the Find a Genetic Counselor database to assist clinicians in locating counselors near their practice.[6] Physicians who connect with geneticists and genetic counselor teams in their local area can call on these consultants as needed to field family history questions, obtain current testing guidelines, and assist in the education of their office staff who may be screening family histories and offering initial education about available genetic counseling and testing services.

Web-based genetic resources for clinicians are also easily accessible for professional understanding of state-of-the-art science and to obtain patient education materials, which are downloadable for distribution. GeneReviews, GeneTests, and

GeneClinics are online resources developed at the University of Washington and funded by the National Institutes of Health.[7] The site provides comprehensive current summaries of most genetic conditions (GeneReviews) along with a list of testing centers (GeneTests), and contact information for genetic professionals throughout the country (GeneClinics). Physicians searching for patient education material may wish to contact their local genetic counseling center, as well as explore pamphlets available for purchase from the American College of Obstetrics and Gynecology. The March of Dimes maintains downloadable patient education materials available in Spanish.[8] Other reputable sites maintain similar content for professional and patient education (eg, Genetics Home reference http://ghr.nlm.nih.gov/).[9]

OBSTETRICIAN GYNECOLOGISTS AS PRIMARY GENETIC COUNSELORS

Physicians recognize genetic risk for the patient and most often initiate the genetic counseling process. These early explanations of risk, including options for genetic testing and in turn, suggestions for referral to genetic consultants, can be considered primary genetic counseling. Indeed, women look to their obstetrician gynecologist as a trusted advisor, and take careful stock of the explanations and suggestions made by the physician. For this reason, physician opinions about controversial topics (such as prenatal screening for Down syndrome) often register with patients and may influence their perception of testing options. Women expect to obtain medical advice from their physicians, but in the arena of genetic testing, decision making is often fraught with ethical and moral implications, with divergent opinions possible between the physician, the patient, and the patient's family members. Skilled clinicians recognize the importance of offering education and options while maintaining personal neutrality in the patient's choices around genetic information. These initial conversations lay important groundwork for the patient referred to formal genetic counseling.

REFERRAL TO GENETIC SERVICES

Genetic professionals are trained to perform comprehensive risk assessment, teach patients about genetic mechanisms, and communicate the risk and testing options in a way that is meaningful to the patient. Counseling skills explore the patient's personal interpretation of genetic information and the implications for family members. Genetic counselors seek to reach a level of engagement such that the patient can reflect in her own words an accurate understanding of her genetic situation and personal rationale for why she does or does not want to pursue further testing. Genetic counseling sessions typically last 30 minutes for a brief encounter, 60 minutes for a routine encounter, and 90 to 120 minutes for complex cases such as an initial cancer genetic counseling session. This level of engagement is beyond what could typically be offered by the physician in a busy practice and provides the opportunity to focus on the patient's understanding of her situation as she makes decisions regarding genetic health issues. Consultations are typically billed as office visits or consults, under Current Procedural Terminology (CPT) coding guidelines.[10] Increasingly, genetic counselors bill for their work under CPT code 96,040, initiated in 2007 to describe the unique work of the Master of Science–prepared genetic counselor.

Physicians who refer to genetic counseling are asked to provide at minimum the indication for referral and significant family or medical history, along with pertinent laboratory results. Genetic professionals expect to provide the physician with a complete summary of the consultation including who was present, pertinent family history for 3 generations, the genetic risk assessment, testing offered, patient uptake of testing, and test results along with a follow-up plan, if indicated. Often, genetic centers provide a consultation summary directly to the patient as well, as documentation of genetic counseling and test results that may be pertinent to the patient or her family members in the future.

GENETIC COUNSELING IN OBSTETRICS AND GYNECOLOGY

Each stage of the life cycle has potential genetic risk for the female patient. Progressing from the reproductive years to later adulthood, the following sections outline current genetic counseling indications. Several of these topics are explored in depth in other articles in this issue and the reader is encouraged to explore these articles as noted.

Preconception

Women seeking preconception care are provided with information from their physician for health promotion (eg, nutrition counseling) and risk reduction (eg, smoking cessation). The preconception period is the ideal time for genetic risk assessment. The gynecologist is encouraged to use this opportunity to explore family medical history for potential genetic risk to offspring. Several standard family history questionnaires have been designed to identify most indications for further genetic evaluation including those available through the American College of Obstetricians and Gynecologists (ACOG). Patients can also be encouraged to complete an online family history. For example, the Surgeon General's office recently created a genetic history tool in a form amenable for inclusion in an electronic medical record.[11] The preconception visit is also a good time to review other risk factors, such as infection/immunization history and review of medications for potential teratogenicity with prescription revision if necessary.

Ancestry-based Carrier Screening

Preconception and early pregnancy are an appropriate time to broach ancestry-based carrier testing with the patient and her partner. Genetic histories elicited should include countries of ancestry. The obstetrician gynecologist is encouraged to look beyond the obvious. Most Americans have more than 1 country of origin within their heritage and will need to be specifically questioned to accurately elicit potential carrier risk. Although whites are often of European descent, ancestries with risk factors beyond cystic fibrosis are not uncommon. Similarly, African Americans and Asian Americans with multiple lineages will be ascertained when questioned carefully. Ancestry-based risk such as that associated with Ashkenazi Jewish heritage and others will not necessarily be identified by the patient herself; the careful practitioner may wish to use a family medical history tool that elicits detailed ancestry.

Current practice guidelines for ancestry carrier screening are available from ACOG and ABMG.[12–14] Carrier screening for hemoglobinopathies, cystic fibrosis (see the article by Jeffrey S. Dungan elsewhere in this issue for further exploration of this topic), and Jewish genetic disease (see the article by Klugman and Gross elsewhere in this issue for further exploration of this topic) are relatively well established clinically. Physicians and their office staff who counsel patients should be familiar with identifying at-risk populations, explaining carrier frequencies as well as autosomal recessive inheritance, and the specificity of the carrier screen as part of an informed consent process. Documentation of patient education and uptake or declination of carrier testing should be included in the medical record.

Genetic counselors are available to counsel patients identified as carriers of a recessive trait and to further evaluate the risk status of the partner. During pregnancy, expedited genetic counseling referral is indicated so that an at-risk couple can be identified, counseled, and offered appropriate prenatal diagnosis within the gestational age for chorionic villus sampling or amniocentesis. Genetic counselors may also be asked to educate physician office staff in identifying ancestry-based risk, offering appropriate carrier testing, and facilitating informed consent within the physician's practice.

As carrier testing guidelines evolve, physician practice evolves. Carrier screening for SMA is an example of new capabilities for identifying genetic risk (see the article by Thomas W. Prior elsewhere in this issue for further exploration of this topic). New tests added to the genetic screening list present a challenge to the physician to deliver enough education to facilitate informed consent without overwhelming the patient. Genetic counselors can facilitate incorporating screening by educating staff and care providers. Formal genetic counseling is currently recommended before carrier screening for SMA.

Prenatal Screening and Diagnosis

ACOG guidelines from 2007 provide detailed direction for developing prenatal screening and diagnosis strategies within an obstetrics practice.[15,16] Genetic professionals in the local practice area may provide first trimester screening, multiple marker screening, and/or a variety of combined and contingency screening models available in addition to prenatal diagnosis via chorionic villus sampling and amniocentesis. Alternatively, obstetricians in areas without local genetic counseling services may interface with a genetic counselor liaison at a national reference laboratory to develop a plan. Obstetricians are encouraged to use genetics professionals for assistance in designing their approach to prenatal screening and diagnosis, and especially for developing an education and consent process for their patients. Genetic counselors are typically available on request to educate office staff who provide initial education to patients, and facilitate the transfer of screen-negative and screen-positive results to the patient. For example, multiple marker screening has become a routine aspect of prenatal care, yet the consent process and in particular, the delivery of screen-positive results to the patient, often occurs without careful consideration.[17]

Targeted ultrasound of fetal anatomy as a second trimester screening tool can identify an unexpected need for genetic evaluation and counseling. In an otherwise normal pregnancy, the finding of fetal anomaly(ies) creates anxiety for parents and a management problem for the obstetrician. Maternal fetal medicine specialists working with genetic professionals can assist, by providing an evaluative approach to identify etiology, predict outcome, discuss potential interventions, and assist the patient and her partner in making decisions about pregnancy management. Diagnostic procedures may include routine cytogenetic evaluation via amniocentesis, and increasingly includes integration of new techniques for identifying genomic imbalance, such as microarray technologies (see the article by Fruhman and Veyver elsewhere in this issue for further exploration of this topic). Given the development of fetal intervention protocols in several centers, the maternal fetal genetics team can also consider evolving treatment opportunities with the family. The genetic counselor can provide emotional support in what is often a crisis for the family, and extend that support to the delivery and beyond. The genetic counselor will ensure the patient is referred to appropriate resources for continuing care after birth, such as local pediatric genetic or multispecialty care clinics and local and national support resources.

Abnormal Prenatal Diagnosis

Genetic counseling is always indicated following abnormal prenatal diagnosis via chorionic villus sampling or amniocentesis. Ideally, preprocedure counseling by the obstetrician, maternal fetal medicine specialist, and/or genetics professional has explored parent perspectives on prenatal diagnosis and the possibility of an abnormality. Regardless, the reality of diagnosis creates a new situation and preprocedure statements as to how a couple would manage an affected pregnancy are often revised following a prenatal diagnosis.

As test results are finalized, the obstetrician and genetics professional should create a mutual plan for delivering information to the pregnant couple. Recall studies have suggested guidelines for relaying abnormal diagnoses: to speak to the patient as soon as possible, preferably with her partner present, in a place in which they feel comfortable such as their home and/or at a prearranged time.[18] This initial alert to the diagnosis is typically by telephone and should be followed by in-person consultation within a short period. In addition to the counseling session, written and online resources for further exploration of the situation should be provided, as well as the opportunity for the patient to communicate with parents who have raised a child with the condition and those who have chosen pregnancy termination or adoption.

The referring obstetrician may choose to contact the patient personally, at home when the couple are likely to be together. Alternatively, the obstetrician may ask the genetic counselor to deliver the diagnosis. In either case, the family should ideally be seen for genetic counseling within a 24-hour period to review genetic etiology, diagnostic features, and the natural history of the condition using current reference materials. Discussion of potential pregnancy outcome choices may include pregnancy termination, releasing the newborn for adoption, or planning for the delivery and care of the child with the genetic condition. Genetic counselors will connect these parents with appropriate resources for further education about the condition. Genetic counselors strive to provide care without coercion or specific interest in the outcome of the pregnancy. As such, their counseling skills can be used to assist in facilitating the patient's thought process and to navigate potential couple disagreement as the parents evaluate their choices. Genetic counselors can also connect the patient with others who have worked through similar dilemmas, as well as local and national support resources.

Coordination of care through the remainder of the pregnancy is crucial for the patient with an abnormal prenatal diagnosis. The genetic counselor can assist the obstetrician in supporting the patient in her decision, and continue that support through the remainder of the pregnancy. Genetic counselors often provide long-term support at anticipated critical times; for example, as the patient who terminated an affected pregnancy approaches her expected due date, the genetic counselor may telephone the patient to provide supportive care in her grief process. Care may also extend into subsequent pregnancies, which regardless of recurrence risk estimates, typically are associated with great anxiety for parents who have previously experienced an abnormal outcome.

Multiple Pregnancy Loss, Infertility and Assisted Reproduction

For the patient who has experienced multiple pregnancy loss or infertility, genetic evaluation to rule out or establish a cause is routine. This may include cytogenetic evaluation of fetal tissues from spontaneous abortion, particularly that of the third or greater loss for the patient. Aneuploidy, a common cause of spontaneous loss, may also portend increased risk in subsequent pregnancy, depending on the findings. Structural rearrangements identified in fetal tissue or through parental peripheral blood chromosome analysis often indicate significant recurrence risk and may have familial risk implications. The genetic counselor serving as laboratory liaison can alert the obstetrician to the risk and suggest appropriate follow-up. Formal genetic counseling should be offered in cases of identified chromosome abnormality, to include review of the etiology, recurrence risk, future pregnancy testing options, and to explore the patient's psychosocial experience with loss, including providing referral to support resources.

Thrombophilia as a cause for multiple pregnancy loss is a complex area of obstetrics care for which prophylactic treatment holds promise (see the article by Walker and Gregg elsewhere in this issue for further explanation of this topic). Several of the thrombophilias include inherited mutations predisposing the patient to clotting events. Genetic counseling to promote patient understanding of the condition, as well as to identify other family members at risk for thrombophilic events is indicated. Some tertiary medical centers have developed thrombophilia clinics where multispecialty care can be provided to the patient and family members. Thrombophilia evaluation in obstetrics and gynecology is an example of integration of mutation analysis with medical treatment to promote healthy outcomes, a form of personalized medical care.

The multiple causes of infertility include genetic causes for some couples. Rare couples will be identified in which 1 member has a structural chromosomal rearrangement. Women with infertility caused by a genetic diagnosis such as Turner syndrome or other X chromosome abnormality are indicated for genetic counseling and potentially assisted reproduction. Couples undergoing in vitro fertilization (IVF) with intracytoplasmic sperm injection should be counseled about the potential increased risk for aneuploidy and other birth defects. Male factor infertility evaluation typically includes chromosome analysis and Y factor studies to rule out common genetic causes.[19] The reproductive endocrinologist typically initiates these evaluations and refers to genetic counseling as appropriate. Increasingly, couples undergoing IVF are offered preimplantation genetic diagnosis for single gene disorders, inherited chromosomal translocations, and aneuploidy. Genetic counseling for assisted reproduction has evolved with genetic counselors providing input to the American Society of Reproductive Medicine to develop guidelines for genetic evaluation.[20]

Women's Health Beyond the Reproductive Years

In middle adulthood, premature ovarian failure may present and require genetic evaluation as a component of the work-up. Peripheral blood cytogenetic tests are indicated to identify chromosomal conditions such as structural abnormalities in the X chromosome. More recently, the association of the Fragile X premutation carrier state with premature menopause suggests that molecular carrier testing for Fragile X syndrome be considered (see the article by Lee P. Shulman elsewhere in this issue for further exploration of this topic). Given the familial implications of Fragile X, pretest genetic counseling is indicated.

Cancer management for women with premenopausal diagnoses of breast or ovarian cancer, or those with a significant family history of these and other cancers, has evolved to include genetic testing with counseling about risk reduction options for mutation-positive patients (see the article by Lee P. Shulman elsewhere in this issue for further exploration of this topic). As part of the cancer management team, a genetic counselor can elicit cancer-sensitive family history, ascertain appropriate medical records and pathology documentation of cancer diagnoses, and provide pre- and posttest counseling for breast/ovarian, several colorectal syndromes, and other cancers with identified genetic predisposition. The focused process of meeting with a cancer genetic counselor before testing allows the patient and referring gynecologist to be assured that the implications of testing are considered and the most appropriate test ordered. Cancer genetics as a subspecialty is rapidly evolving, as are testing guidelines; a cancer genetics professional can be of great assistance to the gynecologist seeking current information.

Just as cancer represents an illness with complex etiology, other conditions with complex genetic and environmental interplay are becoming better understood. This unfolding is happening rapidly in cardiology. Multiple mutations integral to cardiac function have been identified and understanding their role in heart disease holds promise for improved treatments in the future. For example, hypertrophic cardiomyopathy is usually caused by inherited mutations of 1 or more genes that code for heart muscle proteins. Genetic testing can be diagnostic and provide risk estimates for family members, including those who may be at risk for sudden cardiac death.[21] Genetic counseling for cardiac disease is a growing subspecialty, and for women with a family history of early onset heart disease, it may offer hope for intervention.

FUTURE POTENTIAL WITHIN PERSONALIZED MEDICINE

Several subspecialties within medicine can expect further elucidation of genetic factors in the near future. Several clinical trials are underway and others in design for treatment based on mutation analysis. Research-based genetic counselors, often serving as study coordinators, are in the midst of this translational activity. One example is ongoing clinical trials of an experimental drug for cystic fibrosis that is targeted to a specific type of genetic mutation in the cystic fibrosis gene that affects about 10% of individuals with the disease.[22] Future medical prescription will likely include a growing evidence base of treatment defined by molecular characterization of the condition. This era of personalized medicine will eventually include many areas of health care, and is a research effort to be monitored for its potential medical impact.

SUMMARY: THE OBSTETRIC GENETIC CONNECTION

Genetic counseling is a specialty service integrally related to obstetrics and gynecology. This article discusses the genetic counseling resources available to the obstetrician gynecologist, including contact with referral centers near their practice and web-based resources for current genetic information. Many practice guidelines related to genetics have been generated to assist the physician, who is the primary genetic counselor for the patient, identifying risk and introducing genetic testing options that sometimes include referral to formal genetic counseling. Genetic counselors and geneticists are available resources for the obstetrician for education about state-of-the-art genetic services, including research-based interventions, and as direct care providers, serving as a consultant to the physician. As genetics continues its integration into a more personalized, mutation-based medical approach, the author encourages obstetrician gynecologists to forge relationships with genetics professionals for assistance in navigating this evolving and exciting area of medicine.

REFERENCES

1. American Board of Medical Genetics. Available at: http://www.abmg.org/pages/training_specialties.shtml. Accessed November 30, 2009.
2. American Board of Genetic Counseling. Available at: http://www.abgc.net/English/view.asp?x=1. Accessed November 30, 2009.
3. Resta R, Biesecker BB, Bennett RL, et al. A new definition of genetic counseling: National Society of Genetic Counselors task force report. J Genet Couns 2006;15: 77–83.
4. National Society of Genetic Counselors. Available at: http://www.nsgc.org/about/AnnualReport08/Membership.cfm. Accessed December 1, 2009.

5. Edwards JA. Transnational approach: a commentary on Lost in translation: limitations of a universal approach in genetic counseling. J Genet Couns 2009. DOI:10.1007/s10897-009-9260-x.

6. National Society of Genetic Counselors. Available at: http://www.nsgc.org/source/Members/cMemberSearch.cfm. Accessed November 30, 2009.

7. Uhlmann WR, Guttmacher AE. Key Internet genetic resources for the clinician. JAMA 2008;299(11):1356–8.

8. March of Dimes. Available at: http://www.marchofdimes.com/pnhec/4439_4140.asp. Accessed December 28, 2009.

9. Genetic Home Reference. Available at: http://ghr.nlm.nih.gov. Accessed January 19, 2010.

10. American Medical Association. Available at: http://www.ama-assn.org/ama/pub/physician-resources/solutions-managing-your-practice/coding-billing-insurance/cpt.shtml. Accessed December 1, 2009.

11. Surgeon General's Family Health History. Available at: https://familyhistory.hhs.gov/fhh-web/home.action. Accessed November 30, 2009.

12. Gross SJ, Pletcher BA, Monaghan KG. Carrier screening in individuals of Ashkenazi Jewish descent. Genet Med 2008;10(1):54–6.

13. ACOG Committee on Practice Bulletins. ACOG Committee Opinion No. 442: Preconception and prenatal carrier screening for genetic diseases in individuals of Eastern European Jewish descent. Obstet Gynecol 2009;114:950–3.

14. Pletcher BA, Gross SJ, Monaghan KG, et al. The future is now: carrier screening for all populations. Genet Med 2008;10(1):33–6.

15. ACOG Committee on Practice Bulletins. ACOG Practice Bulletin No. 77: screening for fetal chromosome abnormalities. Obstet Gynecol 2007;109(1):217–27.

16. ACOG Committee on Practice Bulletins. ACOG Practice Bulletin No. 88: invasive prenatal testing for aneuploidy. Obstet Gynecol 2007;110(6):1459–67.

17. Kobelka C, Mattman A, Langlois S. An evaluation of the decision-making process regarding amniocentesis following a screen-positive maternal serum screen result. Prenat Diagn 2009;29(5):514–9.

18. Skotko BG, Kishnani PS, Capone GT, et al. Prenatal diagnosis of Down Syndrome: how to best deliver the news. Am J Med Genet A 2009;149:2361–7.

19. Stahl PJ, Masson P, Mielnik A, et al. A decade of experience emphasizes that testing for Y microdeletions is essential in American men with azoospermia and severe oligozoospermia. Fertil Steril 2009. DOI:10.1016/j.fertnstert.2009.09.006.

20. American Society of Reproductive Medicine. Available at: http://www.asrm.org/Patients/topics/genetics.html. Accessed December 29, 2009.

21. Chang JJ, Lynm C, Glass RM. Hypertrophic cardiomyopathy. JAMA 2009;302(15):1720.

22. National Institutes of Health. Study of Ataluren in cystic fibrosis. Available at: http://www.clinicaltrials.gov/ct2/show/NCT00803205?term=ataluren+for+cystic+fibrosis&rank=1. Accessed December 29, 2009.

Newborn Screening for Treatable Genetic Conditions: Past, Present and Future

Susan Hiraki, MS[a], Nancy S. Green, MD[b],*

KEYWORDS

• Newborn screening • NBS • Genetic screening
• Obstetrician-gynecologist

Newborn screening (NBS) is a public health mandate in each state, with the goal to reduce the morbidity and mortality of particular congenital conditions. Since its inception in the mid-1960s, NBS has evolved into a complex public health system, linking blood sampling in newborn nurseries with testing by state or other centralized laboratories, complex notification and follow-up systems involving public health, hospitals, and primary and specialty medical care. The development of new testing technologies and therapies, the expansion of screening panels, the widespread adoption of NBS across the country, oversight from state and federal entities, input from family and commercial entities, and the emergence of new social and ethical issues related to screening are all factors that contribute to the why, what, and how of NBS. Successful implementation of this multilevel system depends on involvement of different health professionals. Of particular importance in this review is the pivotal role of the obstetrician-gynecologist.

THE ROLE OF THE OBSTETRICIAN/GYNECOLOGIST

The increasing complexity of screening test panels and treatments, as well as the myriad of medical, ethical, and logistical issues, requires the participation of health care professionals who can effectively convey key information to their patients. At the interface between pre- and postnatal care, obstetrician-gynecologists are uniquely positioned to present critical information to families at the ideal time: before and just following delivery. Communication about NBS during routine prenatal care is

Funding: none.
[a] Mailman School of Public Health, Columbia University, 722 West 168 Street, New York, NY 10032, USA
[b] Department of Pediatrics, Columbia University Medical Center, PO Box 168, Black Building 2-241, 630 West 168 Street, New York, NY 10032, USA
* Corresponding author.
E-mail address: nsg11@columbia.edu

a well-established practice recommendation of the American College of Obstetrics and Gynecology (ACOG),[1] and by the federal Human Resources and Service Administration[2] and key national entities such as the American Academy of Pediatrics (AAP),[3] the American College of Medical Genetics (ACMG),[4] March of Dimes,[5] and others. To assist primary care providers in responding to NBS results, ACMG has developed "Fact Sheets" for communicating with families and for determining appropriate follow-up of infants with positive screening results (http://www.acmg.net/resources/policies/ACT/condition-analyte-links.htm) (**Fig. 1**).

HISTORY OF NBS

Phenylketonuria (PKU), discovered in 1934, was recognized as a disorder of inborn error of metabolism resulting in toxicity from excessive blood phenylalanine levels, causing mental retardation and other irreversible neurologic damage.[6] Recognizing the need for early detection of the disorder in newborns, in 1963 Guthrie and Susie developed a methodology to screen for this disorder using a few drops of blood collected on a filter paper,[6] which would detect elevated phenylalanine levels in infants and thereby identify those with PKU.[7] Early identification allowed for initiation of treatment in the neonatal period to prevent the otherwise inevitable clinical manifestations of PKU. PKU soon became the paradigm for population-based genetic screening. However, the benefits of early detection and treatment of PKU were accompanied by an unanticipated challenge for prenatal care. Affected women became more likely to reach reproductive age and successfully give birth to genetically unaffected children. This success has led to the next generation's risk of maternal PKU and the teratogenic effect of hyperphenylalanemia on fetal brain, heart, and growth.[8] Today, refinement of guidelines for the management of maternal PKU has resulted in considerably fewer adverse outcomes.[9]

In addition to testing for disorders such as congenital hypothyroidism, hemoglobinopathies and galactosemia, use of tandem mass spectrometry (MS/MS) has made possible the screening of up to 55 disorders with a single assay. MS/MS is effective for screening for particular metabolic disorders via precise measurement of specific amino acids and other analytes in blood to detect amino acid, organic acid, and fatty acid disorders.[10] In addition, most states are now incorporating some degree of DNA-based analysis of specific gene mutations into state NBS testing, such as in confirmation of cystic fibrosis (CF).

NBS TODAY

The Human Genome Project and other large-scale advances in genomics have enhanced the potential to identify an expanding range of disorders in the presymptomatic period.[11] Further identification of disease-causing genes and the refinement of these techniques promise a continued increase in the number of conditions that can be tested for in newborns.[12] Expansion of test panels increases the number of children protected from risk of major disability and death. Combining advances in new technologies and knowledge about the disorders and treatments with extensive public health commitment and advocacy has led all states to offer NBS for PKU and more than 50 different disorders. NBS programs also exist in much of the developed world. Although most of the disorders are rare, the combined incidence of all the screened disorders is estimated to be as high in 1 in every 500 to 1000 births (**Table 1**).[13]

Newborn screening is a state-based program, and although all states have legislation for newborn screening, states have varied widely in their screened conditions. In

Newborn Screening ACT Sheet
[Primary TSH test/Elevated TSH]
Congenital Hypothyroidism

Differential Diagnosis: Primary congenital hypothyroidism (CH); transient CH.

Condition Description: Lack of adequate thyroid hormone production.

You Should Take the Following Actions:

- Contact family **IMMEDIATELY** to inform them of the newborn screening test result.
- Consult pediatric endocrinologist; referral to endocrinologist if considered appropriate.
- Evaluate infant (see clinical considerations below).
- Initiate timely confirmatory/diagnostic testing as recommended by the specialist.
- Initiate treatment as recommended by consultant as soon as possible.
- Educate parents/caregivers that hormone replacement prevents mental retardation.
- Report findings to state newborn screening program.

Diagnostic Evaluation: Diagnostic tests should include serum **free T4** and **thyroid stimulating hormone (TSH)**; consultant may also recommend **total T4 and T3 resin uptake**. Test results include **reduced free T4 and elevated TSH** in primary hypothyroidism; if done, **reduced total T4 and low or normal T3 resin uptake**.

Clinical Considerations: Most neonates are asymptomatic, though a few can manifest some clinical features, such as prolonged jaundice, puffy facies, large fontanels, macroglossia and umbilical hernia. Untreated congenital hypothyroidism results in developmental delay or mental retardation and poor growth.

Additional Information:
(Click on the name to take you to the website. Complete URLs are listed in the Appendix)
New England Newborn Screening Program

American Academy of Pediatrics

Genetics Home Reference

Referral (local, state, regional and national):
Lawson Wilkins Pediatric Endocrine Society "Find a Doc"

Contact local/regional University-affiliated medical center

Fig. 1. ACT sheet for hypothyroidism. ACT sheets follow a similar format for all conditions. ACT sheet content enables care providers to address patient and family needs while seeking expert consultation. (*From* American College of Medical Genetics; with permission.)

the past few years, national recommendations providing guidance for screening programs and local advocacy efforts have helped bring states up to minimum standards,[3–5] such that all states currently universally screen their neonates for at least 21 core disorders.[5] Differences between programs remain, with some states screening for as many as 54 conditions. In addition to variability in testing targets,

Table 1
Incidence of selected disorders

Selected Disorders	Incidence (Live Births)	Confirmed Cases Reported (Out of 4.4 Million Infants Screened)
Biotinidase deficiency	1/61,000	158
Congenital adrenal hyperplasia	1/15,000	241
Cystic fibrosis	1/31,000 to 1/3200	619[a]
Galactosemia (classic)	1/30,000	106
Homocystinuria	1/200,000 to 1/335,000	4
Sickle cell anemia	>1/5000	1583
Phenylketonuria (classic)	1/26,000 to 1/200,000	162
Congenital hypothyroidism	>1/5000	1982
Maple syrup urine disease	1/185,000	19
Medium-chain acyl-CoA dehydrogenase deficiency (MCAD)	1/4900 to 1/17,000	213
Glutaric aciduria type 1	1/20,000 to 1/40,000	40
	Total	5127

[a] Out of 3.8 million infants screened.
Data from NNSGRC National Newborn Screening Information System (NNSIS), 2008 http://www2.uthscsa.edu/nnsis/menu.cfm; NCBI Gene Tests: Reviews http://www.ncbi.nlm.nih.gov/sites/GeneTests/review?db=GeneTests; Recommended Newborn Screening Tests: 29 Disorders - March of Dimes http://www.marchofdimes.com/professionals/14332_15455.asp.

there is also some variation in how state NBS programs are implemented and the extent of public health follow-up. However, NBS generally follows a process of sample collection, screening, communication, confirmation of diagnosis, and follow-up (**Fig. 2**). In assessing the accuracy of the screening result, external factors such as preterm birth, timing of sample collection, transfusion, diet, and total parenteral nutrition need to be considered (**Table 2**).

In 2006, ACMG published a report funded by the Maternal and Child Health Bureau (MCHB) of the Health Resources and Services Administration (HRSA) that established, for the first time, criteria to evaluate conditions for screening, and identified a universal minimum recommended panel of screenable disorders.[4] The ACMG report was endorsed by ACOG, AAP, and other major professional groups. Based on "the availability of scientific evidence, availability of a screening test, presence of an efficacious treatment, adequate understanding of the natural history of the condition, and whether the condition was either part of the differential diagnosis of another condition or whether the screening test results related to a clinically significant condition,"[2] the ACMG report identified 3 groups of conditions: (1) belonging to the core panel for screening (29 conditions) (**Table 3**); (2) so-called secondary targets: conditions for which screening is not directed but are identified or suggested when screening for the core panel (25 conditions); or (3) disorders deemed not appropriate for NBS because of inadequate screening, diagnostic, or accepted treatment. There is general consensus that newborn screening should be focused on conditions that present reasonably early in childhood, and for which early efficacious treatment is available.[3,14] Another significant step toward the standardization of NBS criteria came with the creation of the federal Advisory Committee on Heritable Disorders in

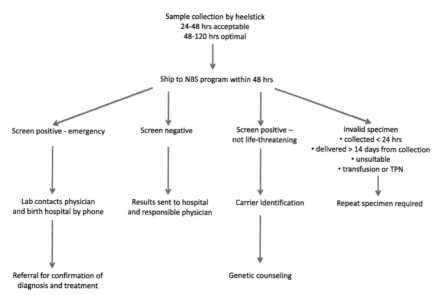

Fig. 2. Flowchart on NBS process. Several states re-screen their infants at two weeks of age. (*Data from* Newborn Screening Program, NYS Department of Health, Wadsworth Center, http://wadsworth.org/newborn/guide.htm. State and Regional Newborn Screening Resources, NNSGRC, http://genes-r-us.uthscsa.edu/resources/newborn/state.htm.)

Newborns and Children (ACHDNC), which is charged with providing advice and recommendations on standards and policies for universal NBS screening tests to the federal department of Health and Human Services (HHS). To take advantage of expanding opportunities generated by new knowledge about disorders, screening and treatments, this HHS advisory committee has created a formal nomination process to expand the universal recommended panel of NBS disorders, including a nomination form that outlines the evidence needed for the consideration of new conditions to be added to the universal panel.[2]

Conditions Tested

The disorders targeted by newborn screening consist primarily of metabolic conditions that can be classified as fatty acid disorders, amino acid disorders, and organic acid disorders. Also included are congenital hypothyroidism, hemoglobinopathies, and other assorted conditions (see **Table 3**).

Fatty acid disorders

Fatty acid oxidation disorders are inherited metabolic conditions that lead to an accumulation of fatty acids and a decrease in cell energy metabolism. Each of these disorders is associated with a specific enzyme defect in the fatty acid metabolic pathway. During periods of prolonged fasting or increased energy demands, these otherwise healthy children can present with vomiting, lethargy, coma, and seizures. They usually have autosomal recessive inheritance. Affected children generally require a frequent food source to avoid a period of relative starvation because they have impaired ability to metabolize fats (see **Table 2**).

Table 2
Influencing factors

Selected Disorders	Factors Influencing the Accuracy of the Test Result	Treatment
Biotinidase deficiency	Transfusion	Biotin replacement
Congenital adrenal hyperplasia	Sample timing	Hormone replacement
Congenital hypothyroidism	Preterm birth	Hormone replacement
Cystic fibrosis	Sample timing, transfusion	Pulmonary disease management, nutritional supplementation
Galactosemia	Diet, transfusion, total parenteral nutrition	Dietary galactose restriction
Homocystinuria	Diet, sample timing, total parenteral nutrition	Dietary protein restriction
MCAD deficiency	Sample timing	Frequent feedings
PKU	Diet, total parenteral nutrition	Dietary phenylalanine restriction
Sickle cell disease/ hemoglobinopathies	Preterm birth	Prophylactic antibiotics, vaccinations, management of symptoms
Tyrosinemia	Diet, preterm birth, total parenteral nutrition	Dietary tyrosine restriction, prevention of fumarylacetoacetate accumulation

Data from GeneTests: Reviews. Available at: http://www.ncbi.nlm.nih.gov/sites/GeneTests/review?db=GeneTests. Accessed November 8, 2009. Kaye CI, Committee on Genetics. Introduction to the newborn screening fact sheets. Pediatrics 2006;118(3):1304–12.

Amino acid disorders

Amino acid disorders are conditions that result in a build up of toxins caused by the inhibition of amino acid metabolism, including PKU. Symptoms have an episodic nature and include poor feeding, lethargy, seizures, developmental regression, hepatomegaly, hypotonia, hyperammonemia, unusual odor, growth failure, mental retardation, and seizures. They usually have autosomal recessive inheritance. Treatment generally consists of a low-protein diet and medications to prevent ammonia buildup (see **Table 2**).

Organic acid disorders

Each organic acid disorder is associated with a specific enzyme deficiency, which leads to the accumulation of blood levels of organic acids. Toxic levels can result in lethargy, vomiting, failure to thrive, developmental delay, liver disease, ataxia, seizures, coma, and hypotonia. These disorders are associated with variable age of onset, depending on the particular condition. Most have an autosomal recessive inheritance and require dietary protein restriction and nutritional supplementation (see **Table 2**).

Hemoglobinopathies

Hemoglobinopathies are conditions in which impaired or abnormal production of hemoglobins result in anemia of variable severity. The primary target of

Table 3
Treatments and factors influencing test accuracy

	Disorders of Metabolism				
Fatty Acid Oxidation	Organic Acid Oxidation	Amino Acid Oxidation	Hemoglobinopathies	Other
Medium-chain acyl-CoA dehydrogenase deficiency	Isovaleric academia	Pheynylketonuria	Sickle cell anemia (Hb S/S)[a]	Congenital hypothyroidism
Very long-chain acyl-CoA dehydrogenase deficiency	Glutaric academia type 1	Maple syrup urine disease	Hb S/β-thalassemia[a]	Biotinidase deficiency
Long-chain 3-OH acyl-CoA dehydrogenase deficiency	3-Hydroxy 3-methyl glutaric aciduria	Homocystinuria	Hb S/C disease[a]	Congenital adrenal hypoplasia
Trifunctional protein deficiency	Multiple carboxylase deficiency	Citrullinemia		Classic galactosemia
Carnitine uptake defect	Methylmalonic academia	Arginosuccinic academia		Cystic fibrosis[a]
	3-Methylcrotonyl-CoA carboxylase deficiency	Tyrosinemia type 1		Hearing loss
	Methylmalonic academia			
	Propionic academia			
	β-Ketothiolase deficiency			

[a] Routine prenatal and neonatal screening offered.
Data from Newborn screening: toward a uniform screening panel and system. Genet Med 2006;8(Suppl 1):1S–252S.

hemoglobinopathy screening is sickle cell anemia and sickle variants (HbSC and sickle-β thalassemia). Hemoglobin abnormalities may result from structural defects in the hemoglobin protein such as sickle cell, insufficient production causing thalassemia, or abnormal pairing of normal hemoglobin proteins. These disorders are most prevalent in populations of Asian, African, Indian, and Mediterranean descent. Treatments include prophylactic penicillin against bacterial infections, as well as vaccinations, medications, and periodic assessments to minimize chronic organ damage from disrupted blood flow (see **Table 2**).

Other

Congenital hypothyroidism Congenital hypothyroidism results from inadequate or absent thyroid hormone causing severe growth and mental retardation. Treatment requires lifelong hormone replacement therapy to prevent mental retardation and growth delay (see **Table 2**).

Congenital adrenal hyperplasia Congenital adrenal hyperplasia is most commonly caused by a deficiency in 21-hydroxylase, resulting in impaired cortisol production. Excessive androgen production can result in virilization of females. Severely affected infants are also at risk for life-threatening salt-wasting. Treatment includes lifelong hormone replacement (see **Table 2**).

Biotinidase deficiency This enzyme deficiency results in frequent infection, hearing loss, seizures, and mental retardation. If untreated, coma and death could result. Treatment involves daily doses of biotin (see **Table 2**).

Galactosemia Deficient galactose-1-phosphate uridyltransferase (GALT) enzyme activity results in impaired galactose metabolism. Features include cataracts, liver failure, mental retardation, infection, and death. Immediate dietary intervention restricting galactose intake improves prognosis, however there is still a risk of developmental delay (see **Table 2**).

Cystic fibrosis CF is caused by mutations in the *CFTR* gene, which regulates ion channel conductance. It is characterized by pulmonary disease, pancreatic dysfunction, and gastrointestinal problems. Treatment depends on severity of symptoms, but often involves management of pulmonary complications and nutritional supplementation, and enzyme therapies to enhance gut absorption and respiratory health (see **Table 2**).

ETHICAL, SOCIAL AND FINANCIAL ISSUES

In some ways, the rapid advancement of newborn screening technology is outpacing the accommodation of ethical and clinical standards. Pertinent issues include consent, sample storage, ethnic disparities, social implications, and funding.

Consent

Currently, most newborn screening programs are mandatory, with the assumption that the minimal risk of screening is outweighed by the significant public health benefits to ensue if a newborn were identified and treated for 1 of these conditions. A presumed parental consent model is based on the paradigm that NBS is considered to be part of routine care. Many states, Canada and the United Kingdom offer an opt-out option (eg, for religious reasons). In the United States, only Maryland and Wyoming require explicit written consent. If identifying a condition had no direct medical benefit for the affected child, if there were no immediacy to initiate treatment, and/or if screening were to identify predisposition for a disorder rather than diagnosis, then a general consensus exists that explicit parental consent should be obtained.[15-17] State programs that pilot expanded NBS, such as in Massachusetts and California, usually require parental consent.[18,19]

Sample Storage and Future Use

The need for storage of residual blood spots continues to be a consideration in improving NBS programs and in the public health and research communities. There is wide variability in the amount of time that state programs retain blood spots, ranging from several weeks to more than 21 years. Sample storage raises issues related to consent, privacy, and confidentiality, as well as logistical challenges pertaining to cost and resources required for storage.[3] Recent federal funding to the ACMG to organize national studies of these rare disorders may increase pressure on state NBS programs to retain residual samples.

Ethnic Disparities

Challenges related to screening in diverse ethnic populations may become more relevant with expanding testing panels, especially as programs expand their screening algorithms to include DNA-based screening. Screening by identification of specific mutations will identify some but not all possible disease-causing mutations. Because some mutations tend to segregate to certain populations, DNA-based tests may exhibit variable levels of sensitivity depending on who is being screened. Hence, issues related to justice and equity may need to be addressed when considering the addition of new testing targets.[20]

Social Implications

In addition to the many clinical benefits offered by NBS, potential benefits to family members include informing reproductive decision-making and the opportunity for financial and psychological preparation of affected families. However, potential social harms may also ensue from the detection of incidental findings, false-positive results, and the identification of asymptomatic carriers. Such implications must be considered before testing and to ensure appropriate follow-up with patients and parents.[20]

Funding

In general, public health programs receive federal funds to be used at the discretion of state policies. Funding sources for NBS vary widely between states, and can be financed through fees paid by Medicaid or other third party payers, health providers, laboratories, hospitals, and parents.[21] Although the additional costs of expanding screening panels may be largely offset by the increased efficiency and lower false-positive rate offered by MS/MS technology,[21] there are increasing concerns about the growing need for resources in the future. Added costs to public health are of particular importance during an era laden with additional pressures on a slim public health infrastructure.

FUTURE DIRECTIONS

Much attention is currently focused on adding new disorders to the recommended universal panel (see **Table 3**). Severe combined immunodeficiency (SCID) is one of the most recent disorders to be considered by the federal advisory committee for inclusion. Already implemented in Wisconsin, much effort has been devoted to developing a feasible and effective method for detection from dried blood spots.[22] If adopted by states, SCID would be the first disorder for which NBS is primarily DNA-based. DNA-based mutation analysis in NBS programs will likely continue to expand to more disorders and more variants. At the extreme, microarray chip technology could become an efficient and specific method of screening for congenital disorders, and at the same time shift NBS from a phenotype-based system to more of a geno-type-based system.[23]

Other evolving aspects of NBS include the prospect of screening for conditions with genetic implications for family health such as Fragile X or Duchenne Muscular Dystrophy, for which no medical treatment is available to improve the health of the affected child. As expansion of knowledge continues to bring new opportunities for medical intervention and improved health, the costs of lifelong treatments are under increasing strain. For example, medical insurance often does not now cover treatments for disorders identified via NBS, even the costly low-protein formulas to treat PKU. Increasingly, attention is being focused on what role, if any, states should play in covering the costs of disorders identified through NBS.

As electronic medical records increasingly become part of integrated health care delivery, routine prenatal and neonatal screening can be linked to provide more organized care for carriers and affected individuals. Priority for linked screening should be given for those disorders that are screened for in the prenatal and newborn periods. For example, prenatal carrier detection of cystic fibrosis or sickle cell should be used to inform NBS about children and families at risk of screenable conditions. Obstetricians can provide the key link to communicating pivotal maternal-infant genetic health issues, reducing confusion and improving maternal-child health. As newborn and prenatal screening for more disorders continues to increase, obstetricians will be needed to provide even better protection for the health of our families.

SUMMARY

Newborn screening is a complex public health program that has been very successful at significantly reducing infant morbidity and mortality from specific genetic conditions. As this program continues to expand, the role of the obstetrician as patient educator has become increasingly important. The need and desire for prenatal education about newborn screening has been demonstrated, and obstetricians are in the prime position to satisfy this vital role.

REFERENCES

1. American College of Obstetricians and Gynecologists. ACOG committee opinion no. 393, December 2007. Newborn screening. Obstet Gynecol 2007;110(6): 1497–500.
2. MCHB - Advisory Committee on Heritable Disorders in Newborns and Children. Available at: http://www.hrsa.gov/heritabledisorderscommittee/. Accessed November 8, 2009.
3. Lloyd-Puryear MA, Tonniges T, van Dyck PC, et al. American Academy of Pediatrics Newborn Screening Task Force recommendations: how far have we come? Pediatrics 2006;117(5 Pt 2):S194–211.
4. Newborn screening: toward a uniform screening panel and system. Genet Med 2006;8(Suppl 1):1S–252S.
5. Recommended newborn screening tests: 29 Disorders - March of Dimes. Available at: http://www.marchofdimes.com/professionals/14332_15455.asp. Accessed November 8, 2009.

6. Fernhoff PM. Newborn screening for genetic disorders. Pediatr Clin North Am 2009;56(3):505–13.
7. Guthrie R, Susi A. A simple phenylalanine method for detecting phenylketonuria in large populations of newborn infants. Pediatrics 1963;32:338–43.
8. Levy HL, Waisbren SE, Güttler F, et al. Pregnancy experiences in the woman with mild hyperphenylalaninemia. Pediatrics 2003;112(6 Pt 2):1548–52.
9. Hoeks MP, den Heijer M, Janssen MC. Adult issues in phenylketonuria. Neth J Med 2009;67(1):2–7.
10. Wilcken B. Ethical issues in newborn screening and the impact of new technologies. Eur J Pediatr N Engl J Med 2003;162(Suppl 1):S62–6.
11. Kenner C, Moran M. Newborn screening and genetic testing. J Midwifery Women's Health 2005;50(3):219–26.
12. Cunningham G. The science and politics of screening newborns. N Engl J Med 2002;346(14):1084–5.
13. Centers for Disease Control and Prevention (CDC). Impact of expanded newborn screening–United States, 2006. MMWR Morb Mortal Wkly Rep 2008;57(37):1012–5.
14. Therrell BL. U.S. newborn screening policy dilemmas for the twenty-first century. Mol Genet Metab 2001;74(1–2):64–74.
15. Laberge C, Kharaboyan L, Avard D. Newborn screening, banking and consent. Gene Expr 2004;2(3):1–15.
16. Pelias MK, Markward NJ. Newborn screening, informed consent, and future use of archived tissue samples. Genet Test 2001;5(3):179–85.
17. Kerruish NJ, Robertson SP. Newborn screening: new developments, new dilemmas. J Med Ethics 2005;31(7):393–8.
18. Feuchtbaum L, Cunningham G. Economic evaluation of tandem mass spectrometry screening in California. Pediatrics 2006;117(5 Pt 2):S280–6.
19. Pass K, Green NS, Lorey F, et al. Pilot programs in newborn screening. Ment Retard Dev Disabil Res Rev 2006;12(4):293–300.
20. Green NS, Dolan SM, Murray TH. Newborn screening: complexities in universal genetic testing. Am J Public Health 2006;96(11):1955–9.
21. Johnson K, Lloyd-Puryear MA, Mann MY, et al. Financing state newborn screening programs: sources and uses of funds. Pediatrics 2006;117(5 Pt 2):S270–9.
22. Baker MW, Grossman WJ, Laessig RH, et al. Development of a routine newborn screening protocol for severe combined immunodeficiency. J Allergy Clin Immunol 2009;124(3):522–7.
23. Green NS, Pass KA. Neonatal screening by DNA microarray: spots and chips. Nat Rev Genet 2005;6(2):147–51.

Spinal Muscular Atrophy: Newborn and Carrier Screening

Thomas W. Prior, PhD

KEYWORDS

• Spinal muscular atrophy • Carrier testing
• Newborn screening • SMN1 • SMN2

Spinal muscular atrophy (SMA) is a common autosomal-recessive neuromuscular disorder caused by mutations in the survival motor neuron (SMN1) gene, affecting approximately 1 in 10,000 live births.[1] The disease is characterized by progressive symmetric muscle weakness resulting from the degeneration and loss of anterior horn cells in the spinal cord and brainstem nuclei. The disease is classified on the basis of age of onset and clinical course. Two almost identical SMN genes are present on 5q13: the SMN1 gene, which is the SMA-determining gene, and the SMN2 gene. The homozygous absence of the SMN1 exon 7 has been observed in most patients and is being used as a reliable and sensitive SMA diagnostic test. Although SMN2 produces less full-length transcript than SMN1, the number of SMN2 copies has been shown to modulate the clinical phenotype. Carrier detection relies on the accurate determination of the SMN1 gene copies. Because SMA is one of the most common lethal genetic disorders, direct carrier dosage testing has been beneficial to many families. The American College of Medical Genetics has recently recommended population carrier screening for SMA.[2] The management of SMA involves supportive and preventive strategies. New treatments based on increasing the expression of full-length SMN protein levels from the SMN2 gene are being investigated and may be dependent on early detection of the disorder, before the irreversible loss of motor neurons. This could potentially be accomplished through a newborn screening program for SMA. This article focuses on the prevention of SMA through population carrier screening and newborn screening as a means of ensuring early intervention for SMA.

CLINICAL FEATURES

The autosomal-recessive disorder proximal SMA (SMA types I, II, and III [MIMs 253300, 253550, and 253400]) is a severe neuromuscular disease characterized by

Department of Pathology, The Ohio State University, 125 Hamilton Hall, 1645 Neil Avenue, Columbus, OH 43210, USA
E-mail address: thomas.prior@osumc.edu

Obstet Gynecol Clin N Am 37 (2010) 23–36
doi:10.1016/j.ogc.2010.03.001
0889-8545/10/$ – see front matter © 2010 Elsevier Inc. All rights reserved.

obgyn.theclinics.com

degeneration of alpha motoneurons in the spinal cord, which results in progressive muscle weakness and paralysis. The weakness is almost always symmetric and progressive. The predominant pathologic feature of autopsy studies of patients with SMA is loss of motoneurons in the ventral horn of the spinal cord and in brainstem motor nuclei. SMA is the second most common fatal autosomal-recessive disorder after cystic fibrosis (CF), with an estimated incidence of approximately 1 in 10,000 live births.[1]

Childhood SMA is subdivided into three clinical groups on the basis of age of onset and clinical course.[3,4] Type I SMA (Werdnig-Hoffmann disease) is characterized by severe, generalized muscle weakness and hypotonia at birth or before 6 months. Death from respiratory failure usually occurs within the first 2 years. Approximately 60% to 70% of SMA patients have the type I disease.[5] Type II children are able to maintain a sitting position unsupported, although they cannot stand or walk unaided. The phenotypic variability exceeds that observed in type I patients, ranging from infants who sit transiently and demonstrate severe respiratory insufficiency to children who can sit, crawl, and even stand with support. Prognosis in this group is largely dependent on the degree of respiratory involvement. Type III SMA (Kugelberg-Welander syndrome) is a milder form, with a later age of onset, and these children all achieve independent walking. The legs are more severely affected than the arms. Some patients lose the ability to walk in childhood, yet others maintain walking until adolescence or adulthood. They also comprise a less fragile group than type II patients with regard to respiratory and nutritional vulnerability. Type III SMA is further subdivided into two groups: type IIIa (onset <3 years of age) and type IIIb (onset at age ≥3 years). Cases presenting with the first symptoms of the disease at the age of 20 to 30 years are classified as type IV, or proximal adult type SMA. The described classification is based on age of onset and clinical course, but it should be recognized that the disorder demonstrates a continuous range of severity. Lastly, although the disease affects both genders equally, there have been reports that the severe type I is more common in females and that females are less affected than males in the milder SMA types.[6,7]

GENETICS

The SMA gene is located within a complex region containing multiple repetitive and inverted sequences (**Fig. 1**).[8] The *SMN* gene (Entrez Gene ID number 6606) comprises nine exons with a stop codon present near the end of exon 7.[9] Two inverted *SMN* copies are present: the telomeric or *SMN1* gene, which is the SMA-determining gene, and the centromeric or *SMN2* gene. The two *SMN* genes are highly homologous, have equivalent promoters,[10,11] and only differ at five base pairs.[8] The base differences are used to differentiate *SMN1* from *SMN2*. The coding sequence of *SMN2* differs (840C>T) from that of *SMN1* by a single nucleotide in exon 7, which does not alter the amino acid but has been shown to be important in splicing. Homozygous mutations of the *SMN1* gene cause SMA. Both copies of the *SMN1* gene are absent in about 95% of affected patients, whereas the remaining patients have nonsense, frameshift, or missense mutations within the gene. The absence of SMN1 can occur by deletion, typically a large deletion that includes the whole gene, or by conversion to SMN2. Although SMA patients have mutations in *SMN1*, they always carry at least one normal copy of *SMN2*, which is partially functional but unable fully to compensate for the deficiency of the *SMN1* protein. There was initially no SMA genotype-phenotype correlation observed because *SMN1* was found to be absent in most patients, regardless of the disease severity. This is caused by the fact that

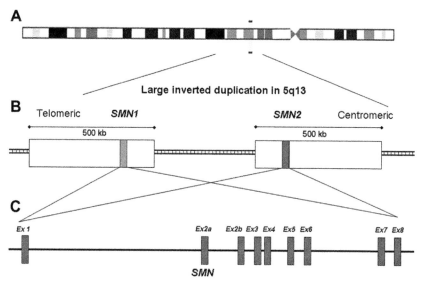

Fig. 1. The *SMN* gene. (*A*) SMA results from mutations in the *SMN* gene located on chromosome 5q13. (*B*) *SMN1* and its centromeric homolog *SMN2* lie with the telomeric and centromeric halves, respectively, of a large inverted 500-kb repeat. (*C*) *SMN* consists of nine exons (1, 2a, 2b, and 3–8) with a stop codon present near the end of exon 7.

routine diagnostic methods do not distinguish between a deletion of *SMN1* and the conversion event whereby *SMN1* is replaced by a copy of *SMN2*. Several studies have now shown that the total *SMN2* copy number modifies the severity of the disease.[12–15] The copy number varies from zero to three copies in the normal population, with approximately 10% to 15% of normal individuals having no *SMN2*. Milder patients with type II or III SMA have been shown, however, to have more copies of *SMN2* than type I patients. Most patients with the severe type I form have one or two copies of genomic *SMN2*, most patients with type II have three genomic *SMN2* copies, and most patients with type III have three or four genomic *SMN2* copies. Three unaffected family members of SMA patients, with confirmed *SMN1* homozygous deletions, were shown to have five copies of genomic *SMN2*.[16] These cases not only support the role of *SMN2* modifying the phenotype, but they also demonstrate that expression levels consistent with five copies of the *SMN2* genes may be enough to compensate for the absence of the SMN1 gene.

This inverse dose relationship between *SMN2* copy number and disease severity has also been supported by the SMA mouse model.[17,18] The SMA mouse models have not only confirmed the susceptibility of motoneuron degeneration to *SMN* deficiency, but have verified that the degeneration can be prevented by increased *SMN2* dosage. Mice lacking the endogenous mouse *Smn* gene, but expressing two copies of the human *SMN2* gene, develop severe SMA and die within 1 week of age; however, mice that express multiple copies of *SMN2* do not develop the disease.

In addition to the *SMN2* copy number, other modifying factors influence the phenotypic variability of SMA. There are very rare families reported in which markedly different degrees of disease severity are present in affected siblings with the same *SMN2* copy number. These discordant sib pairs, which share the same genetic background around the SMA locus, indicate that there are other modifier genes outside the SMA region. Differences in splicing factors may allow more full-length expression from the *SMN2* gene and account for some of the variability observed between discordant sibs.[19] It was also found that in some rare families with unaffected SMN1-deleted females, the expression of plastin 3 (*PLS3*) was higher than in their SMA affected counterparts.[20] PLS3 was shown to be important for axonogenesis and may act as a protective modifier. The identification of gene modifiers not only provides important insight into pathogenesis of SMA, but may also identify potential targets for therapy.

Molecular Pathology

Because all SMA-affected individuals have at least one *SMN2* gene copy, and there are no differences in the amino acid sequence between the two genes, the obvious question that arises is why do individuals with *SMN1* mutations have a SMA phenotype? It has been shown that the *SMN1* gene produces full-length transcript, whereas the *SMN2* gene produces predominantly an alternatively spliced transcript (exon 7 deleted) encoding a protein (SMNΔ7) that does not oligomerize efficiently and is unstable (**Fig. 2**).[21,22] The inclusion of exon 7 in *SMN1* transcripts and exclusion of this exon in *SMN2* transcripts is caused by the single nucleotide difference at +6 in *SMN1* exon 7 (c.840C>T). Although the C to T change in *SMN2* exon 7 does not change an amino acid, it does disrupt an exonic splicing enhancer (ESE) or creates an exon silencer element (ESS), which results in most transcripts lacking exon 7.[23,24] The ESEs and ESSs are *cis*-acting exonic sequences that influence

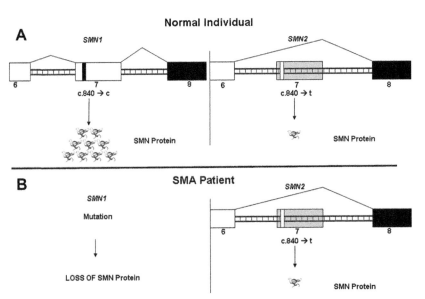

Fig. 2. (*A*) In normal individuals, most full-length SMN transcript and protein is generated from the *SMN1* gene. (*B*) SMA patients have homozygous mutations of *SMN1* but retain at least one copy of the *SMN2* gene. During transcription of *SMN2*, the *SMN2* gene produces predominantly an alternatively spliced transcript (exon 7 deleted) encoding a protein (SMNΔ7), which is unstable. The inclusion of exon 7 in *SMN1* transcripts and exclusion of this exon in *SMN2* transcripts is caused by the single nucleotide difference at +6 in *SMN1* exon 7 (c.840C>T). Small amounts of full-length transcripts generated by *SMN2* are able to produce a milder type II or III phenotype when the copy number of the *SMN2* gene is increased. SMA is caused by low levels of SMN protein, rather than a complete absence of the protein.

the use of flanking splice sites. ESEs stimulate splicing and are often required for efficient intron removal, whereas ESSs inhibit splicing. Whether it is the loss of an ESE or creation of an ESS, the result is a reduction of full-length transcripts generated from *SMN2*. A single *SMN2* gene produces less functional protein compared with a single *SMN1* gene.[25–27] SMA arises because the *SMN2* gene cannot fully compensate for the lack of functional SMN when *SMN1* is mutated. Small amounts of full-length transcripts generated by *SMN2* are able to produce a milder type II or III phenotype, however, when the copy number of the *SMN2* gene is increased. SMA is caused by low levels of SMN protein, rather than a complete absence of the protein.

Finally, a recent report described three unrelated SMA patients who possessed *SMN2* copy numbers that did not correlate with the observed mild clinical phenotypes.[28] A single base substitution in *SMN2* (c.859G>C) was identified in exon 7 in the patients DNA, and it was shown that the substitution created a new ESE element. The new ESE increased the amount of exon 7 inclusion and full-length transcripts generated from *SMN2*, resulting in the less severe phenotypes. The SMA phenotype may not only be modified by the number of *SMN2* genes, but *SMN2* sequence variations can also affect the disease severity. It should not be assumed that all *SMN2* genes are equivalent and sequence changes found within the *SMN2* gene must be further investigated for potential positive or negative effects on *SMN2* transcription.

SMA results from a reduction in the amount of the SMN protein and there is a strong correlation between the disease severity and SMN protein levels.[25,26] The SMN protein is a ubiquitously expressed, highly conserved 294–amino acid polypeptide. The protein is found in both the cytoplasm and nucleus and is concentrated in punctate structures called "gems" in the nucleus.[27] High levels of the protein have been found to exist in the spinal motoneurons, the affected cells in SMA patients. The protein self-associates into a multimeric structures. Biochemically, SMN does not seem to exist within cells in isolation but instead forms part of a large protein complex, the SMN complex. Many of these SMN interacting proteins are components of various ribonuclear protein (RNP) complexes that are involved in distinct aspects of RNA metabolism. The best characterized function of the SMN complex is regulating the assembly of a specific class of RNA-protein complexes, the small nuclear ribonuclear protein (snRNPs).[29] The snRNPs are a critical component of the spliceosome, a large RNA-protein that catalyzes pre-mRNA splicing. SMA may be a disorder resulting from aberrant splicing. Because the SMN protein is ubiquitously expressed, it remains unknown how a loss of a general housekeeping function (snRNP assembly) causes a selective loss of motoneurons in SMA.[30] The high expression of SMN protein in motoneurons may suggest that the neuronal population is more sensitive to decreases in the SMN protein level. The altered splicing of a unique set of premessenger RNAs possibly results in deficient proteins that are necessary for motoneuron growth and survival. In addition to its role in spliceosomal RNP assembly, SMN may have other functions in motoneurons. A subset of SMN complexes are located in axons and growth cones of motoneurons and may be involved in some aspects of axonal transport and localized translation of specific mRNAs.[31,32]

Molecular Diagnostics

The absence of detectable *SMN1* in SMA patients is being used as a reliable and powerful diagnostic test for most SMA patients. The first diagnostic test for a patient suspected to have SMA should be the *SMN1* gene deletion test. The deletion status can be easily tested for by using polymerase chain reaction (PCR) and determining if both copies of SMN1 exon 7 are absent, which is found in about 95% of affected patients. Genetic testing is not only the most rapid and sensitive method to confirm the diagnosis, but the testing allows for further invasive investigations, such as electromyography and muscle biopsy, to be avoided. The SMA deletion test is currently being performed by several diagnostic laboratories and the result can easily be obtained within 1 week. The remaining 5% of affected cases, without the homozygous absence of SMN1 exon 7, are compound heterozygotes having one SMN1 deletion and a small intragenic mutation. When a patient with a SMA clinical phenotype possesses only a single copy of SMN1, it is likely that the remaining SMN1 copy contains a more subtle mutation, including nonsense mutations, missense mutations, splice site mutation insertions, and small deletions. Sequencing the SMN1 gene is required for the detection of the nonhomozygous deletion types of mutations and confirms the diagnosis in most SMA cases (>98%). Unfortunately, sequencing the coding region of SMN1 is performed in only a few diagnostic laboratories. If, however, a patient is shown to possess two copies of SMN1, then other motoneuron disorders should be considered, such as SMA with respiratory distress, X-linked SMA, distal muscular atrophy, and juvenile amyotrophic lateral sclerosis.

NEWBORN SCREENING

The correlation between the SMA phenotype and the SMN2 copy number in SMA patients and the demonstration that sufficient SMN protein from SMN2 in transgenic mice can ameliorate the disease has made the SMN2 gene an obvious target that can be modulated in therapeutic strategies. New treatments based on increasing the expression of full-length SMN protein levels from the SMN2 gene are being investigated. Studies have shown that the SMN2 promoter can be activated and full-length SMN RNA and protein levels increased by several other histone deacetylase inhibitors including phenylbutyrate and valproic acid. Both of these drugs have been in clinical use for many years for other indications and have well established safety profiles in children and consequently are now being used in SMA clinical trials.[33,34] A pilot study of phenylbutyrate showed that the drug was well tolerated.[35] Two small open-label trials of valproic acid have reported modest strength or functional benefit in a subset of type III/IV SMA patients.[36,37] Swoboda and coworkers[38] recently demonstrated that valproic acid can be used safely in SMA patients greater than 2 years of age, as long as carnitine status is closely monitored.

The success of the current clinical trials and treatments in the future may depend on identifying individuals as early as possible, in order to begin the treatment before potentially irreversible neuronal loss. In infants with type I SMA, rapid loss of motor units occurs in the first 3 months and severe denervation with loss of more than 95% of units within 6 months of age.[39] A small window for beneficial therapeutic intervention exists in infants with type I SMA, which may occur before a clinical diagnosis, and therapies need to be administered within the newborn period for maximum benefit. This could potentially be accomplished through a newborn screening program for SMA. Newborn screening would provide an opportunity to initiate therapy before the irreversible organ damage, and to prospectively document the most early disease manifestations. Presymptomatic enrollment into clinical trials may also enhance the possibility of identifying an effective drug intervention, because clinical trials in symptomatic patients with end-stage denervation may not actually show the efficacy of a prospective therapy.

The use of tandem mass spectrometry has greatly expanded the number of disorders screened for in newborn screening laboratories. Tandem mass spectrometry is used to detect disorders of amino acid, organic acid, and fatty acid metabolism and acylcarnitines in a single multiplex assay format from blood spots. The technique has been shown to be rapid, sensitive, and robust and has a high throughput. The identification of SMA patients during the newborn period can only be accomplished by DNA testing for the SMN1 exon 7 homozygous deletion, however, because the disorder does not have a biochemical marker. SMA presents a unique challenge because the testing requires DNA as the substrate, which differs from present tests using tandem mass spectrometry. Direct DNA testing is the next innovation in newborn screening, but currently is used primarily for reflex testing for first-tier positive results (see the article by Hiraki and Green elsewhere in this issue for further exploration of this topic). With its sizeable capacity for multiplexing, array technologies have been touted as the application of choice for the first-tier analysis of DNA in newborn screening.[40,41] Using liquid microbead array for the detection of the homozygous SMN1 exon 7 deletion, Pyatt and coworkers[42] demonstrated that newborn screening for SMA can be accomplished. In a series of blood spots, all 164 affected samples were correctly found to have the homozygous SMN1 deletion, whereas 157 unaffected samples were excluded.[41] The clinical sensitivity of a SMA newborn screen is approximately 95% to 98%, because it does not identify affected individuals who are compound heterozygotes possessing one deleted SMN1 allele and a second allele with a point mutation or the very rare case of a patient with a homozygous point mutation. These individuals are identified during the symptomatic phase, which may be too late for an effective treatment. The families of these children are negatively impacted by a normal newborn screen for SMA, because these children are diagnosed later and do not obtain early intervention.

There is a growing consensus that newborn screening can still be extremely valuable for genetic conditions for which there is not a specific effective treatment, and there are a number of disorders currently screened for that do not respond to treatment. A newborn screening program for SMA would not only allow patients to be enrolled in clinical trials at the earliest time period, but would enable patients to obtain proactive treatment earlier in the disease progression with regard to nutrition, physical therapy, and respiratory care. Many SMA infants show progression in the setting of nutritional compromise. If identified early, this situation could be managed proactively by nutritional interventions. Furthermore, given the availability of noninvasive respiratory treatments, such as mechanically assisted cough devices to facilitate clearing of secretions, early implementation of such interventions may help to reduce respiratory morbidity and extend lifespan. The same types of arguments are used to support newborn screening for CF: earlier intervention and more proactive treatments. It has been reported in observational trials that CF patients identified by newborn screening have better lung function and growth compared with CF patients diagnosed clinically.[43–46] Furthermore, identifying SMA-afflicted individuals at birth eliminates the pain and cost of unnecessary testing that often takes place in attempting to diagnose an affected patient. The results from newborn screening would also be important for the child's family because of the possibility for the prevention of additional cases through genetic counseling and carrier testing of at-risk family members. A newborn screen would provide an early and definite diagnosis, and allow parents to make earlier and informed reproductive choices. A newborn screening program would also identify milder later-onset cases of SMA and their identification may become controversial. The well-documented genotype-phenotype association between the SMN2 copy number and clinical severity, however, may help specifically to select those patients who benefit most from early therapeutic intervention.

CARRIER TESTING

SMA is one of the most common lethal genetic disorders, with an approximate carrier frequency of 1 in 35 for non-Hispanic whites, 1 in 41 for Ashkenazi Jews, 1 in 53 for Asians, and 1 in 117 for Hispanics.[47] SMN1 dosage testing is used to determine the SMN1 copy number and detect SMA carriers: carriers possess one SMN1 copy and noncarriers have two SMN1 copies and occasionally have three SMN1 copies. Carrier detection for the heterozygous state was initially shown to be more technically challenging because the SMA region is characterized by the presence of many repeated elements.[13] It has been observed that the SMN2 copy number fluctuates: approximately 10% to 15% of unaffected individuals lack the SMN2 copy, whereas many of the more mildly affected SMA patients have more copies. A straightforward dosage assay using the SMN2 gene as the internal control would not be reliable. There have now been a number of techniques developed for the detection of SMA carriers, however, including real-time PCR,[6] competitive PCR,[13] competitive PCR with primer extension,[48] Taqman technology,[49] denaturing high-performance liquid chromatography,[50] and multiple ligation-dependent probe amplification.[51]

There are two limitations of the dosage carrier test. First, approximately 2% of SMA cases arise as the result of de novo mutation events,[52] which is high compared with most autosomal-recessive disorders. The high rate of de novo mutations in SMN1 may account for the high carrier frequency in the general population despite the genetic lethality of the type I disease. The large number of repeated sequences around the SMN1 and SMN2 locus likely predisposes this region to unequal crossovers and recombination events and results in the high de novo mutation rate. The de novo mutations have been shown to occur primarily during paternal meiosis.[52] Second, the copy number of SMN1 can vary on a chromosome; it has been observed that about 5% of the normal population possess three copies of SMN1.[13] It is possible for a carrier to possess one chromosome with two copies and a second chromosome with zero copies (**Fig. 3**).[2,13,53] Using haploid conversion technique, which allows for single

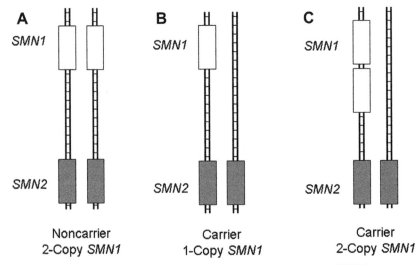

Fig. 3. SMA noncarriers and carriers. (A) A noncarrier has two copies of SMN1, one on each chromosome 5. (B) A SMA carrier has one copy of SMN1 on one chromosome and 0 copies on the other chromosome. (C) A SMA carrier with one chromosome with two SMN1 copies and a second chromosome with zero copies.

chromosome analysis, Mailman and coworkers[54] identified a parent of an affected child with a two-copy chromosome. The finding of two *SMN1* genes on a single chromosome has serious genetic counseling implications, because a carrier with two *SMN1* genes on one chromosome and a *SMN1* deletion on the other chromosome has the same dosage result as a noncarrier with one *SMN1* gene on each chromosome 5 (see **Fig. 3**). The finding of normal *SMN1* copy dosage significantly reduces the risk of being a carrier; however, there is still a residual risk of being a carrier, and subsequently a small recurrence risk of future affected offspring for individuals with 2 *SMN1* gene copies. Genetic counseling is a key process associated with carrier testing, and the concept of residual risk is not new to genetic counselors who regularly discuss residual risk when counseling couples about CF carrier screening. Risk assessment calculations using bayesian analysis are essential for the proper genetic counseling of SMA families.[55] A recent report has shown that there are significant differences in carrier frequencies and the two-copy chromosome genotypes among different ethnic groups.[48] The adjusted risk estimate in the African-American population was shown to be more than five times greater than that of the white population because of the high frequency of the two-copy alleles detected in the African-American population. The results from this study provide adjusted detection rates based on ethnicity, and allow for more accurate bayesian risk estimates.

Population Carrier Screening

In current practice, patients with a family history of SMA are most often tested for carrier status. Because there is a high panethnic carrier frequency,[48] and the carrier test has a relatively good sensitivity (approximately 90%), why has population-based carrier screening not been implemented? One major factor is that the general population is virtually unfamiliar with SMA. Because the affected type I children die within the first 2 years of life, most individuals have little or no exposure or appreciation of the severity of this very common genetic disorder. The American College of Medical Genetics, however, recently recommended panethnic population carrier screening for SMA.[2] The goal of population-based SMA carrier screening is to offer the test to all couples of reproductive age, identify couples at risk for having a child with SMA, and allow couples to make informed reproductive decisions. Ethnic-based carrier screening is currently recommended for a number of other genetic disorders with similar carrier frequencies (eg, Canavan disease, familial dysautonomia, thalassemia). The prototype for ethnic-based carrier screening was testing for Tay-Sachs disease in the Ashkenazi Jewish population, where carrier testing has been offered since 1969. Carrier screening, followed by prenatal diagnosis when indicated, has resulted in a dramatic decrease in the incidence of Tay-Sachs disease in the Jewish population.[56] It is generally accepted that the following criteria should be met for a screening program to be successful: (1) the disorder is clinically severe, (2) a high frequency of carriers in the screened population, (3) availability of a reliable test with a high specificity and sensitivity, (4) availability of prenatal diagnosis, and (5) access to genetic counseling. SMA does meet the criteria cited. The choice to have a SMA carrier test should be made, however, by an informed decision.

Carrier Screening Issues

The American College of Obstetricians and Gynecologists (ACOG) Committee on Genetics recommended against general population preconception and prenatal screening for SMA at this time.[57] There were several issues on which ACOG based its opposition to panethnic carrier screening. One issue that the committee suggests must be addressed before recommending panethnic SMA screening is the development of education materials. There is no question that education for both patients and primary obstetrician-gynecologists is a priority for any successful screening program. Educational brochures are available to both patients and primary obstetrician-gynecologists, however, and provide information about SMA and the inheritance patterns,[58] and several commercial companies also offer educational material. The ACOG committee report also states that pilot studies specific to SMA have to be completed to determine patient preference and best practices relative to patient counseling. Although the ACOG report makes no mention of CF, for which ACOG has recommended population-based carrier screening since 2002, using CF as a comparison may help to provide answers to several of the issues raised by the ACOG report. CF does have a higher carrier frequency of 1 in 25 for non-Hispanic whites than SMA (1 in 35 for non-Hispanic whites), but both diseases are still relatively common and have the same inheritance pattern. Furthermore, SMA is the leading genetic cause of death in infants under 2 years of age. There were funded CF pilot programs, however, which addressed several of the ACOG issues raised, including feasibility, cost effectiveness, and patient's preference in regards to carrier screening. In general, these pilot studies demonstrated that most Americans welcome carrier screening and the knowledge such screening provides.[59] Although it is true that pilot studies have not been conducted specific to SMA carrier screening, the existing CF studies have broad application and involve many of the same principals for SMA carrier screening.

Lastly, ACOG indicates that panethnic carrier screening for SMA should wait until a cost-effectiveness analysis is investigated. If cost-effectiveness is a primary determining factor for inclusion of a disorder in a carrier screening program, then diseases that are fatal in early childhood and have no treatment would be excluded from screening because of low costs of care associated with the disease. This represents a monumental shift in thinking. Historically, important criteria for inclusion in a carrier screening program have been diseases that are most often fatal in early childhood and do not have a treatment or cure.

Formal genetic counseling services must be made available to anyone requesting this testing. Because the counseling system already exists for CF in most settings, it should be possible to add counseling specific for SMA without too much difficulty. It is important that all individuals undergoing testing understand that a carrier is a healthy individual who is not at risk of developing the disease but has a risk of passing the gene mutation to his or her offspring. It is also important that individuals undergoing carrier testing recognize that the test does not provide genotype-phenotype information. There is no question that the lack of predicting an accurate phenotype makes the counseling more complex. This is also the case for CF, for which carrier screening has been recommended in the prenatal setting in the United States since 2001.[59,60] It is difficult to accurately predict if a carrier couple is at risk for having a severe or mildly affected child with CF. Family planning options are available to parents and include egg or sperm donation, adoption, preimplantation genetic testing, and termination of pregnancy. It is imperative that individuals understand the limitations of the molecular testing: two *SMN1* genes in *cis* on the one chromosome 5, presence of rare de novo mutations, and the nondeletion mutations. The issue of these false-negative results must be explained to all individuals undergoing carrier testing. It has been found that the information necessary for individuals to make an informed decision regarding carrier testing can be presented effectively and efficiently through a counseling session enhanced by printed educational material. As is true for carrier screening programs, the testing must be voluntary and occur after informed consent and ensurance of confidentiality is absolutely necessary.

SUMMARY

As a result of the discovery of the SMN gene and elucidation of the mutational spectrum, clinical diagnostic testing for SMA has significantly improved. Until an effective treatment is found to cure or arrest the progression of the disease, prevention of new cases through accurate diagnosis and carrier and prenatal diagnosis is of the utmost importance. The goal of population-based SMA carrier screening is to identify couples at risk for having a child with SMA, allowing carriers to make informed reproductive choices. In the future, newborn screening for SMA may become a reality and allow for the implementation of more proactive treatments. Even though a specific therapy for SMA is not currently available, a newborn screening test may allow a child to be enrolled in a clinical trial before irreversible neuronal loss occurs and allow for relatives to make earlier reproductive decisions. A newborn screening test also removes the clinical uncertainty and unnecessary, costly, and burdensome diagnostic work-up. With the advancement of new technologies and genetic information, it seems certain that there will be additional tests added to the menus of both newborn and universal carrier screening programs. The implementation of these expanded programs will require a new level of support in genetic services for the public.

ACKNOWLEDGMENTS

The author thanks Scott Bridgeman for his assistance with this article.

REFERENCES

1. Pearn J. Incidence, prevalence, and gene frequency studies of chronic childhood spinal muscular atrophy. J Med Genet 1978;15:409–13.
2. Prior TW. Carrier screening for spinal muscular atrophy. Genet Med 2009;10: 20–6.
3. Munstat TL, Davies KE. International SMA consortium meeting. Neuromuscul Disord 1992;2:423–8.
4. Zerres K, Rudnik-Schoneborn S. Natural history in proximal spinal muscular atrophy: clinical analysis of 445 patients and suggestions for a modification of existing classifications. Arch Neurol 1995;52:518–23.
5. Meldrum C, Scott C, Swoboda KJ. Spinal muscular atrophy genetic counseling access and genetic knowledge: parents perspective. J Child Neurol 2007;22: 1019–26.
6. Feldkotter M, Schwarzer V, Wirth R, et al. Quantitative analysis of SMN1 and SMN2 based on real-time LightCycler PCR: fast and highly reliable carrier testing and prediction of severity of spinal muscular atrophy. Am J Hum Genet 2002;70: 358–68.
7. Alias L, Bernal S, Fuentes-Prior P, et al. Mutation update of spinal muscular atrophy in Spain: molecular characterization of 745 unrelated patients and identification of four novel mutations in the SMN1 gene. Hum Genet 2009;125:29–39.
8. Lefebvre S, Burglen L, Reboullet S, et al. Identification and characterization of a spinal muscular atrophy-determining gene. Cell 1995;80:155–65.
9. Burglen L, Lefebvre S, Clermont O, et al. Structure and organization of the human survival motor neuron (SMN) gene. Genomics 1996;32:479–82.
10. Monani UR, McPherson JD, Burghes AHM. Promoter analysis of the human centromeric and telomeric survival motor neuron genes (SMNC and SMNT). Biochim Biophys Acta 2007;1445:330–6.

11. Echaniz-Laguna A, Miniou P, Bartholdi D, et al. The promoters of the survival motor neuron gene (SMN) and its copy (SMNc) share common regulatory elements. Am J Hum Genet 1999;64:1354–70.
12. Campbell L, Potter A, Ignatius J, et al. Genomic variation and gene conversion in spinal muscular atrophy: implications for disease process and clinical phenotype. Am J Hum Genet 1997;61:40–50.
13. McAndrew PE, Parsons DW, Simard LR, et al. Identification of proximal spinal muscular atrophy carriers and patients by analysis of SMNT and SMNC gene copy number. Am J Hum Genet 1997;60:1411–22.
14. Wirth B, Herz M, Wetter A, et al. Quantitative analysis of survival motor neuron copies: identification of subtle SMN1 mutations in patients with spinal muscular atrophy, genotype-phenotype correlation, and implications for genetic counseling. Am J Hum Genet 1999;64:1340–56.
15. Mailman MD, Heinz JW, Papp AC, et al. Molecular analysis of spinal muscular atrophy and modification of the phenotype by SMN2. Genet Med 2002;4:20–6.
16. Prior TW, Swoboda KJ, Scott HD, et al. Homozygous SMN1 deletions in unaffected family members and modification of the phenotype by SMN2. Am J Med Genet A 2004;130:307–10.
17. Hsieh-Li HM, Chang JG, Jong YJ, et al. A mouse model for spinal muscular atrophy. Nat Genet 2000;26:66–70.
18. Monani UR, Coovert DD, Burghes AHM. Animal models of spinal muscular atrophy. Hum Mol Genet 2000;9:2451–7.
19. Hoffman Y, Lorson CL, Stamm S, et al. Htra2-beta 1 stimulates an exonic splicing enhancer and can restore full-length SMN expression to survival motor neuron 2 (SMN2). Proc Natl Acad Sci U S A 2000;97:9618–23.
20. Oprea GE, Krober S, McWhorter ML, et al. Plastin 3 is a protective modifier of autosomal recessive spinal muscular atrophy. Science 2008;320:524–7.
21. Lorson CL, Androphy EJ. An exonic enhancer is required for inclusion of an essential exon in the SMA-determining gene SMN. Hum Mol Genet 2000;9: 259–65.
22. Lorson CL, Hahnen E, Androphy EJ, et al. A single nucleotide in the SMN gene regulates splicing and is responsible for spinal muscular atrophy. Proc Natl Acad Sci U S A 1999;96:6307–11.
23. Cartegni L, Kraniner AR. Disruption of an SF2/ASF-dependent exonic splicing enhancer in SMN2 causes spinal muscular atrophy in the absence of SMN1. Nat Genet 2002;30:377–84.
24. Kashima T, Manley JL. A negative element in SMN2 exon 7 inhibits splicing in spinal muscular atrophy. Nat Genet 2003;34:460–3.
25. Lefebvre S, Burlet P, Liu Q, et al. Correlation between severity and SMN protein level in spinal muscular atrophy. Nat Genet 1997;16:265–9.
26. Coovert DD, Le TT, McAndrew PE, et al. The survival motor neuron protein in spinal muscular atrophy. Hum Mol Genet 1997;6:1205–14.
27. Liu Q, Fischer U, Wang F, et al. The spinal muscular atrophy gene product, SMN, and its associated protein SIP1 are in a complex with spliceosomal snRNP proteins. Cell 1997;90:1013–21.
28. Prior TW, Krainer AR, Hua Y, et al. A positive modifier of spinal muscular atrophy in the SMN2 gene. Am J Hum Genet 2009;85:408–13.
29. Yong J, Wan L, Dreyfuss G. Why do cells need an assembly machine for RNA-protein complexes? Trends Cell Biol 2004;14:226–32.
30. Monani UR. Spinal muscular atrophy: a deficiency in a ubiquitous protein; a motor neuron-specific disease. Neuron 2005;48:885–96.

31. Zhang HL, Pan F, Hong D, et al. Active transport of the survival motor neuron protein and the role of exon-7 in cytoplasmic localization. J Neurosci 2003;23: 6627–37.

32. Rossoll W, Jablonka S, Andreassi C, et al. Smn, the spinal muscular atrophy-determining gene product, modulates axon growth and localization of beta-actin mRNA in growth cones of motoneurons. J Cell Biol 2003;163:801–12.

33. Chang JG, Hsieh-Li HM, Jong YJ, et al. Treatment of spinal muscular atrophy by sodium butyrate. Proc Natl Acad Sci U S A 2001;98:9808–13.

34. Brichita L, Holker I, Huang K, et al. In vivo activation of SMN in spinal muscular atrophy carriers and patients treated with valproate. Ann Neurol 2006;59:970–5.

35. Brahe C, Vitali T, Tiziano FD, et al. Phenylbutyrate increases SMN gene expression in spinal muscular atrophy patients. Eur J Hum Genet 2005;13:256–9.

36. Weihl CC, Connolly AM, Pestronk A. Valproate may improve strength and function in patients with type III/IV spinal muscular atrophy. Neurology 2006;67:500–1.

37. Tsai LK, Yang CC, Hwu WL, et al. Valproic acid treatment in six patients with spinal muscular atrophy. Eur J Neurol 2007;14:e8–9.

38. Swoboda KJ, Scott CB, Reyna SP. Phase II open label study of valproic acid in spinal muscular atrophy. PLoS One 2009;4:e5268.

39. Swoboda KJ, Prior TW, Scott CB, et al. Natural history of denervation in SMA: relation to age, SMN2 copy number, and function. Ann Neurol 2005;57:704–12.

40. Green NS, Pass KA. Neonatal screening by DNA microarray: spots and chips. Nat Rev Genet 2005;6:147–51.

41. Saxena A. Issues in newborn screening. Genet Test 2003;7:131–4.

42. Pyatt RE, Mihal DC, Prior TW. Assessment of liquid microbead arrays for the screening of newborns for spinal muscular atrophy. Clin Chem 2007;53:1879–85.

43. Dankert-Roelse JE, Merelle ME. Review of outcomes of neonatal screening for cystic fibrosis versus non-screening in Europe. J Pediatr 2005;147(3):S15–20.

44. Khoury MJ, McCabe LL, McCabe ER. Population screening in the age of genomic medicine. N Engl J Med 2003;348:50–8.

45. Sims EJ, McCormick J, Mehta A, et al. Newborn screening for cystic fibrosis is associated with reduced treatment intensity. J Pediatr 2005;147:306–11.

46. Siret D, Bretaudeau G, Branger B, et al. Comparing the clinical evolution of cystic fibrosis screened neonatally to that of cystic fibrosis diagnosed from clinical symptoms: a 10-year retrospective study in a French region (Brittany). Pediatr Pulmonol 2003;35:342–9.

47. Hendrickson BC, Donohoe C, Akmaev VR, et al. Differences in SMN1 allele frequencies among ethnic groups within North America. J Med Genet 2009;46: 641–4.

48. Gerard B, Ginet N, Matthijs G,, et al. Genotype determination at the survival motor neurone locus in a normal population and SMA carriers using competitive PCR and primer extension. Hum Mutat 2000;16:253–63.

49. Anhuf D, Eggermann T, Rudnik-Schoneborn S, et al. Determination of SMN1 and SMN2 copy number using Taqman technology. Hum Mutat 2003;22:74–8.

50. Su Y-N, Hung C-C, Li H, et al. Quantitative analysis of SMN1 and SMN2 genes based on DHPLC: a highly efficient and reliable carrier-screening test. Hum Mutat 2005;25:460–7.

51. Huang C-H, Chang Y-Y, Chen C-H. Copy number analysis of survival motor neuron genes by multiplex ligation-dependent probe amplification. Genet Med 2007;9:241–8.

52. Wirth B, Schmidt T, Hahnen E. De novo rearrangements found in 2% of index patients with spinal muscular atrophy: mutational mechanisms, parental origin,

mutation rate and implications for genetic counseling. Am J Hum Genet 1997;61: 1102–11.

53. Ogino S, Leonard DG, Rennert H, et al. Genetic risk assessment in carrier testing for spinal muscular atrophy. Am J Med Genet 2002;110:301–7.

54. Mailman MD, Hemingway T, Darsey RL, et al. Hybrids monosomal for human chromosome 5 reveal the presence of a spinal muscular atrophy (SMA) carrier with two SMN1 copies on one chromosome. Hum Genet 2001;108:109–15.

55. Ogino S, Wilson RB. Genetic testing and risk assessment for spinal muscular atrophy. Hum Genet 2002;111:477–500.

56. Kaback MM. Screening and prevention in Tay-Sachs disease: origins, update, and impact. Adv Genet 2001;44:253–65.

57. ACOG Committee Opinion. Spinal muscular atrophy. Obstet Gynecol 2009; 113(5):1194–6.

58. Claire Altman Heine Foundation. Prevention of spinal muscular atrophy. Available at: http://www.preventsma.org. Accessed December 1, 2009.

59. ACOG Committee Opinion. Update on carrier screening for cystic fibrosis. Obstet Gynecol 2005;106(6):1465–8.

60. Morgan MA, Driscoll DA, Mennuti MT, et al. Practice patterns of obstetrician-gynecologists regarding preconception and prenatal screening for cystic fibrosis. Genet Med 2004;6:450–5.

Ashkenazi Jewish Screening in the Twenty-first Century

Susan Klugman, MD[a,b,*], Susan J. Gross, MD[a,c]

KEYWORDS

- Ashkenazi Jewish genetic screening • Carrier screening
- Jewish genetic disorders

Ashkenazi Jewish (AJ) genetic screening has expanded significantly in the past 4 decades. Individuals of eastern European (Ashkenazi) Jewish descent are at increased risk of having offspring with particular genetic diseases that have significant morbidity and mortality. In addition, there are some disorders, such as cystic fibrosis (CF), for which northern European Caucasians are at comparable risk with those of an AJ background. Carrier screening for many of these Jewish genetic disorders has become standard of care. As technology advances, so does the number of disorders for which screening is available. Thus, we need to continue to be cognizant of informed consent, test sensitivity, confidentiality, prenatal diagnosis, preimplantation genetic screening, and public health concerns regarding testing.

HISTORY OF JEWISH POPULATIONS AND GENETIC EFFECTS

The Jewish people have a history spanning more than 2000 years.[1] They are a migratory people and have established communities throughout the world. Three groups of Jews have been defined by their location of origin: Sephardic Jews (initially from Spain and later predominately northern Africa, the Balkans, Turkey, Lebanon, and Syria), Middle Eastern Jews (from Israel, Iraq, and environs) and Ashkenazi Jews (primarily of eastern European origin). Jews consider themselves a people because of their common religion, dialect, customs, and marriage within the community. Thus, they have maintained a group identity as well as a genetic identity.[2] Many studies have shown that contemporary Jews share several chromosome markers and polymorphisms as well as genetic mutations.[3–5] However, there is no such thing as a Jewish

---

[a] Obstetrics and Gynecology and Women's Health, Albert Einstein, College of Medicine, Bronx, NY, USA
[b] Reproductive Genetics, Montefiore Medical Center, 1695 Eastchester Road, Suite 301, Bronx, NY 10461, USA
[c] Obstetrics and Gynecology, North Bronx Healthcare Network, Bronx, NY, USA
* Corresponding author. Reproductive Genetics, 1695 Eastchester Road, Suite 301, Bronx, NY 10461.
E-mail address: sklugman@montefiore.org

Obstet Gynecol Clin N Am 37 (2010) 37–46
doi:10.1016/j.ogc.2010.01.001
0889-8545/10/$ – see front matter © 2010 Elsevier Inc. All rights reserved.

obgyn.theclinics.com

genome and Jews are more likely to share sequences with fellow non-Jews than with each other.[2]

Current estimates of the world's Jewish population total 13 million, with the overwhelming majority in the United States and Israel. Most individuals of Jewish ancestry in North America are of Ashkenazi origin.[6] Although there are disorders of significance in the non-AJ Jewish population, they are beyond the scope of this article. Testing in the non-AJ community remains limited at this time in the United States but for more information, the reader is directed to the review by Zlotogora and colleagues,[7] which provides information and links to relevant databases.

Founder Effects and Historical Origins

Many of the disorders in the AJ population can be attributed to mutations presumed to have each arisen in a single individual many centuries ago. This phenomenon had been coined the "founder effect"[8] or "genetic drift." This phenomenon can occur when an individual with a relatively rare mutation moves with a small group to a new location and subsequently proceeds to undergo a significant population expansion. The once rare mutation will now be quite common in this new well-defined population group. The same effect can be seen if an individual with a relatively rare mutation is part of a group that is reduced from a once large population to a small group because of loss of members. Again, a once rare mutation will no longer be rare as the denominator (the total members in the group) has now severely contracted. Historically, Jews fell into both categories, as they were often forced to move to new locations or to endure pogroms that greatly lessened their numbers. Using molecular and bioinformatic tools, some investigators have even managed to determine the connection between some of these disorders and historical events in Jewish history.[2] The founder effect is not limited to the AJ population and likely accounts for the higher rate of Tay-Sachs disease (TSD) in French Canadians, although different mutations account for the disease in this population.

HISTORY OF JEWISH GENETIC SCREENING AND TESTING

The history of Jewish genetic screening and testing begins with screening for TSD. The first prenatal detection of TSD was accomplished in 1969.[9] A British ophthalmologist, Warren Tay, in 1881 as well as an American neurologist, Bernard Sachs, originally described the disease in 1887. Both physicians described a fatal disorder that presented in infancy with blindness, loss of motor function, and cerebral degeneration. Klenk, a German professor, in the 1940s reported the metabolic abnormality in TSD affected gangliosides, a new class of lipids. In the next several decades, the underlying defect in lysomal hexsaminidase A activity was elucidated thereby allowing testing of heterozygotes with somewhat decreased enzyme activity.

In the early 1970s, physicians in several predominantly Jewish neighborhoods went door-to-door and collaborated with Jewish community groups to educate and screen Jewish women.[10] Tay-Sachs was known to be of autosomal recessive inheritance whereby carriers were considered silent. Through education and community consultation, the stigma of being labeled a carrier was overcome and was such a success that children diagnosed with Tay-Sachs within the Jewish community have become a rarity to the extent that most children currently diagnosed with TSD are not of Jewish background do not have other identifiable risk factors.[11,12] Proposed mechanisms include unknown AJ ancestry, lack of screening, or laboratory or physician error.

In the early 1980s, Dor Yeshorim, also called The Committee for Prevention of Genetic Diseases, was started in the Ultra Orthodox community. This program advocates anonymous testing, which is performed primarily on young adults. Those tested are given a special number and when 2 individuals contemplate marriage they contact Dor Yeshorim and are informed if their offspring would be at risk. This system has received some criticism but remains popular and has been effective in the Ultra Orthodox community.

Like Tay-Sachs, the Jewish genetic diseases that are screened for today are of autosomal recessive inheritance. Thus, both parents must be carriers and they would not be aware of their carrier status without testing, as carriers do not have any symptoms. Screening does exist for several autosomal dominant disorders seen more frequently in Ashkenazi Jews, such as torsion dystonia,[13] familial breast and ovarian cancer, and familial colon cancer.[14] However, because of the complexity of screening, penetrance, and serious implications for other immediate family members, individual genetic testing is recommended for those at high risk for these disorders and testing is not currently performed during the routine prenatal visit.

Today, many Jewish women are screened in pregnancy for TSD and some of the other Jewish genetic disorders. However, preconception counseling is the ideal time for education and testing so that women have the broadest reproductive options available. Presently, existing barriers to preconception screening include provider education and sufficient time in a busy obstetric practice. Cost of testing may also be an issue as carrier testing for all the disorders can be expensive, potentially hundreds to thousands of dollars. Not all young people have insurance and some may have insurance that does not cover prenatal genetic testing outside of pregnancy. However, some insurance companies do cover preconception genetic testing when couples are seriously contemplating pregnancy.

THE JEWISH GENETIC DISORDERS

Jewish genetic diseases are rare, with an incidence of 1/900 to 1/40,000. However, approximately 1/5 Ashkenazi Jews will be a carrier for 1 of these disorders and approximately one-third of couples will have at least 1 carrier.[15] Sensitivity for carrier testing for these disorders remains high as laboratories are screening for 1 to 4 founder mutations per disorder.

Testing for Jewish genetic diseases has become more readily available and has rapidly expanded in the later half of this decade. Thus, the recommendations for testing and inclusion of certain disorders are also changing beyond TSD alone. In October 2009, the American College of Gynecology and Obstetrics (ACOG), through their Committee on Genetics, reconfirmed their previous recommendation to include TSD, Canavan disease (CD), CF, and familial dysautonomia (FD).[16] In their committee opinion, ACOG added that individuals of AJ descent may inquire about the availability of carrier screening for other disorders such as mucolipidosis IV (MLIV), Niemann-Pick disease type A (NPD-A), Fanconi anemia group C (FA-C), Bloom syndrome (BS), and Gaucher disease (GD).

The American College of Medical Genetics (ACMG) had previously recommended in 2008 that carrier screening be offered for TSD, CD, CF, FD, FA-C, NPD-A, BS, MLIV, and GD to all Jews of AJ background following a conference at which medical professionals and Jewish community groups shared a platform.[15,17] The decision to include disorders beyond those required in the ACOG panel was based on the fact that some of the diseases have devastating outcomes (such as NPD-A) and more importantly, all have excellent detection rates with currently available technologies. Furthermore, broad testing has strong backing from the Jewish community.[17]

Both guidelines do share many elements in common, including individuals with a positive family history should be offered carrier screening and may benefit from genetic counseling. Also recommended in both documents is the importance of testing the Jewish partner even if only 1 member of a couple is of AJ background. Even though the non-AJ partner may not benefit from mutation testing specific to the AJ population, a geneticist can arrange for other testing, such as biochemical testing in the case of TSD or complete gene sequencing for other disorders, to determine if the individual is also a carrier of a specific disorder. Screening for other Jewish genetic diseases, such as glycogen storage disorder type 1A, maple syrup urine disease, dihydrolipoamide dehydrogenase deficiency, familial hyperinsulinism, nemaline myopathy, and Usher syndromes type I and III, are being routinely offered by providers and encouraged by laboratories that are not currently recommended by either the ACMG or ACOG.[18–24] The disease prevalence of these 7 disorders is much less than TSD, CD, CF, and FD. Thus, the detailed discussion in this article is limited to those disorders for which prenatal screening is recommended by ACOG and/or ACMG (**Table 1**).

TSD (ACOG and ACMG)

TSD is a neurodegenerative disorder that presents in the first year of life and is fatal in early childhood. It is caused by a deficiency in β-hexosaminidase A (Hex A) which in turn causes accumulation of a cell membrane glycolipid, Gm2 ganglioside, within the lysosome. Infants are classically macrocephalic because of storage material accumulation in the brain and have the characteristic cherry red spot on their macula. The incidence of TSD is 1:3000, with a carrier frequency of approximately 1:30.[16] As previously mentioned, screening programs initiated in the 1970s have been widely successful, and have led to at least a 90% reduction in the incidence of TSD. Screening is based on a biochemical assay, whereby the actual Hex A enzyme is measured. As protein levels rather than ethnic-specific mutations are being analyzed, biochemical screening is an excellent test regardless of genetic background. Measurement in serum is particularly cost-effective; however, these levels in serum are altered in pregnancy and oral contraceptive use and can lead to excessive inconclusive reports. Therefore, in pregnancy or for women on birth control pills, leukocyte or platelet assay is preferred.[25,26] DNA-only screening tests for the 3 most common mutations has previously been suggested as an alternative to biochemical testing in the AJ population, identifying 93% to 99% of carriers.[27,28] However, these studies were done in a relatively homogeneous AJ population. A recent analysis of TSD by Schneider and colleagues[26] in a population of self-identified AJ individuals concluded that Hex A enzyme levels were crucial in screening for this disorder as more than 10% of carriers would be missed using DNA only. With increasing intermarriage rates and diversity within the population, the National Tay-Sachs & Allied Diseases Association has confirm this recommendation in its 2009 position statement that biochemical and not DNA testing is preferred in this population.[29]

CD (ACOG and ACMG)

CD is also a progressive neurodegenerative leukodystrophy. Onset appears within the first few months of life and is uniformly fatal in early childhood. The disease is caused by a deficiency of aspartoacylase, which leads to accumulation of N-acetylaspartic acid in the brain and urine. Infants have macrocephaly and seizures and the associated pathologic finding is spongy degeneration of the brain.[30] Kronn and Oddoux[31] suggested testing among Ashkenazi Jews in 1995 after a pilot program at New York University revealed a carrier rate in Ashkenazi Jews similar to that of TSD.

Table 1
Characteristics of AJ genetic diseases for which carrier testing is recommended

Disease Name	Major Clinical Characteristics	Carrier Frequency	No. of Mutations Tested	Detection Rate	Carrier Risk After Negative Result[c]
Tay-Sachs Disease	Enzyme deficiency, progressive neurologic disorder, death by age 4 y	1/30	3	94–98[a]	1/484 to 1/1451
Canavan Disease	Progressive neurologic disorder, death in childhood although some survive longer	1/40	2	98	1/2000
Cystic Fibrosis	Lung and gastrointestinal disorders, median survival 30+ y	1/29	5–7	97	1/1000
Familial Dystautonomia	Abnormal sensory and autonomic nervous system functioning, symptomatic treatment only	1/32	2	99	1/3101
Fanconi Anemia Type C	Deficient bone marrow development and function. Rarely reach adulthood	1/89	1	99	1/8801
Niemann-Pick Type A	Storage disorder, mental and physical degeneration. Death by age 2 y for type A	1/90	3	95	1/1781
Bloom Syndrome	Skin, and growth abnormalities, cancer predisposition, death in young adulthood	1/100	1	95–97	1/1981 to 1/3301
Mucolipidosis IV	Lipid accumulation, eye issues, mental retardation	1/127	2	95	1/2521
Gaucher Disease	Storage disorder, enlarged spleen, liver, anemia, bone pain. Life expectancy and severity varies. Enzyme therapy available	1/15	4	95[b]	1/281

[a] Varies based on enzyme versus mutation analysis.
[b] May include homozygous asymptomatic individuals.
[c] Calculated using Bayesian statistical method.

The disease incidence is 1:6400, with a carrier frequency of 1:40.[16] Carrier screening is based on identification of either of the 2 most common mutations in the Ashkenazi population, and has a detection rate up to 98%.

CF (ACOG and ACMG)

CF is a chronic debilitating disease affecting many organ systems, including the lungs, gastrointestinal tract, sweat glands, and the male reproductive tract. It is the most common single gene disorder in Caucasians. CF is caused by a mutation in the gene on chromosome 7 that encodes a protein called the CF conductance transmembrane regulator (CFTR), which in turn regulates the function of chloride channels. More than 1000 mutations have been identified in CFTR. The severity of disease is variable. Treatment is available and includes pancreatic enzymes, respiratory therapy, nutrition, and aggressive management of infection.[32]

In 2001, ACMG and ACOG introduced guidelines for prenatal and preconception carrier screening for CF and recommended that screening be offered to high-risk couples, such as Caucasians (including Ashkenazi Jews) who are planning a pregnancy. In 2005, ACOG reconfirmed these guidelines and introduced the concept of pan ethnic screening as most obstetricians were indeed offering CF screening to women of all backgrounds.[33] Amongst AJ individuals, the disease incidence of CF ranges from 1:2500 to 1:3000, with a carrier frequency of 1:29. The common AJ mutations are included in the ACOG recommended screening panel and therefore adhering to ACOG guidelines will identify approximately 97% of CF mutations.

FD (ACOG and ACMG)

Patients with FD have a sensorimotor neuropathy, resulting in inadequate development of the sensory and autonomic systems, which results in significant gastrointestinal reflux, lung disease, decreased pain and temperature perception, absence of tears and blood pressure abnormalities. FD presents in infancy and occurs almost exclusively in the AJ population. Carrier screening was recommended by ACOG in 2004.[34] Treatment includes supportive care of all systems affected and can improve survival.[35] The disease incidence for FD is 1:3600 with a carrier frequency of 1:32.[16] Two mutations accounts for more than 99% of the mutations in the AJ people, however 1 mutation is responsible for most carriers.[36] Greater than 99% of carriers and greater than 99% of affected fetuses can be identified.

FD-C (ACMG)

FD-C is characterized by progressive bone failure, congenital anomalies (absent thumbs, radial hypoplasia, cardiac, renal, gastrointestinal, and neurologic abnormalities) and a predisposition to malignancy. FD-C is caused by a propensity to chromosome breakage and increased sensitivity to DNA cross-linking agents. Onset is variable, ranging from birth to 9 years. Patients can be treated with stem cell transplantation however median survival is only until the late teenage years.[37]

FD-C has an incidence of 1:32,000 and a carrier frequency in Ashkenazi Jews of 1:89.[16] A single mutation is most commonly responsible in Ashkenazi Jews, and has not been found in any affected individual of non-Jewish ancestry. Screening would identify more than 99% of carriers.

NPD-A (ACMG)

Like Tay-Sachs, NPD-A is a progressive neurodegenerative disease with onset in infancy and fatal in early childhood. It is caused by a deficiency of sphingomyelinase resulting in an accumulation of sphingomyelin in the lysosome. Infants present with hepatosplenomegaly, hypotonia, and feeding issues. Cherry red spots are seen in the macula of half of the patients.[38] NPD-A has an incidence of 1:32,000 and a carrier frequency in the AJ population of 1:90.[16] Three mutations account for approximately 95% of mutations in the AJ people.

BS (ACMG)

BS is a chromosomal instability disorder that presents in infancy and is characterized by short stature, impaired intellect, photosensitivity, and immunodeficiency. These patients have a predisposition to cancer, commonly leukemia and gastrointestinal malignancy. The median age of death is 28 years.[39] BS is extremely rare in the general population, but has an incidence of 1:40,000 in Ashkenazi Jews with a carrier frequency of 1:100.[16] A complex frameshift mutation accounts for more than 99% of the mutations in the AJ population.

MLIV (ACMG)

Like TSD, MLIV is a lysosomal storage disease that is characterized by growth delays, severe mental retardation, and ophthalmologic abnormalities. This disease is caused by abnormal membrane endocytosis resulting in accumulation of lipids and mucopoly-saccharides in the lysosome. Patients present early in childhood with developmental delay, intellectual impairment, and eye issues (corneal clouding and retinal degeneration). They can have a normal life span, however, most affected patients never attain language or motor function past the capacity of a 2-year-old.[40] The incidence of disease is 1:62,500 and the carrier frequency in the AJ population is 1:127.[16] Two mutations account for more than 95% of mutant alleles in Ashkenazi Jews. Screening would detect approximately 95% of carriers.

GD (ACMG)

GD is also a lysosomal storage disorder caused by a deficiency in glucocerebrosidase resulting in an accumulation of glucosylceramide in the macrophages of the reticulo-endothelial system of the liver, spleen, bone marrow, and lungs. It is subdivided into 3 types. Type 1, which has a wide range of expression, is the most common type found in Ashkenazi Jews. Onset may begin in early childhood and be characterized by bone fractures, hepatosplenomegaly, and thrombocytopenia. Many cases are mild or asymptomatic, and approximately half do not present until the age of 45 years. The average life expectancy is estimated to be 68 years.[41] GD is the most prevalent genetic disorder amongst Ashkenazi Jews with an incidence of 1:900, and a carrier frequency of 1:15.[16] Screening is based on the 4 most common mutations and detects approximately 95% of carriers. Some have questioned routine screening for this disorder because of the variable expression of the disease, the possibility of identifying asymptomatic affected individuals, and the availability of enzyme replacement therapy for management of the disease.[42] However, there can be very significant morbidity associated with GD, including bone fractures in young people. Furthermore, therapy is available but can be associated with significant cost. In addition, there is considerable support for screening within the community and families dealing with GD.[17]

CURRENT RECOMMENDATIONS

- Ideally, screening should occur before conception.
- A general description of the disorders should be provided. Detailed descriptions of the particular disorders are not necessary and if a carrier is identified, such

discussions can take place at that time for the particular disorder in question. Audiovisual materials to help with overall education of couples are certainly appropriate.

- Individuals should be made aware that carriers are healthy and 1 in 5 people of AJ background will be a carrier.
- Ensure that there is an understanding of residual risk; no matter how good the test, there is a small possibility with DNA testing that a mutation is missed.
- If only 1 member of a couple is of AJ decent, that person should be tested first.
- If someone has a Jewish grandparent, testing is warranted.
- Formal genetic counseling should be facilitated if desired by an individual or if felt necessary by the obstetrician or health care provider.
- When a carrier is identified, this information has great import to the entire family. However, as explicitly stated in the ACOG guidelines,[16] the individual should be encouraged to contact family members. There is no provider-patient relationship with the relatives and confidentiality must be respected.

SUMMARY

Prenatal care providers must be aware of the current recommendations for AJ genetic testing as put forth by ACOG. The ACMG recommendations are similar to those of ACOG in that both groups recommend testing for TSD, CD, CF, and FD. However, although ACOG states the patient may inquire about testing for FA-C, NPD-A, BS, MLIV, and BS, ACMG recommends screening. Providers must be able to recognize situations for which genetic counseling and/or prenatal diagnosis and/or preimplantation genetic screening would be appropriate. As technology advances and becomes more accurate and cost-effective, screening for even more disorders may be available in the future. Because TSD is no longer seen predominantly in the AJ community, it can be considered a disorder of the general population, albeit rare, with a carrier rate of approximately 1/300. However, despite this rare carrier frequency, there are calls from this community for pan ethnic screening. Although currently not recommended, screening for disorders once considered Jewish genetic diseases may one day become part of the obstetrician's practice in the future as genetic knowledge continues to expand and marriage between racial and ethnic groups likewise can be expected to increase in the future.

REFERENCES

1. Scheindlein R. A short history of the Jewish people – from legendary times to modern statehood. New York: Oxford University Press; 1998.
2. Ostrer H. A genetic profile of contemporary Jewish populations. Nat Rev Genet 2001;2:891–8.
3. Livshits G, Sokal RR, Kobyliansky E. Genetic affinities of Jewish populations. Am J Hum Genet 1991;49(1):131–46.
4. Nebel A, Filon D, Brinkmann B, et al. The Y chromosome pool of Jews as part of the genetic landscape of the Middle East. Am J Hum Genet 2001;69(5): 1095–112.
5. Motulsky AG. Jewish diseases and origins. Nat Genet 1995;9:99–101.
6. Mandell L. Berman National Jewish population survey. Available at: http://www.jewishdatabank.org/national.asp. Accessed January 20, 2010.
7. Zlotogora J, van Baal S, Patrinos GP. The Israeli National Genetic Database. Isr Med Assoc J 2009;11(6):373–5.

8. Mayr E. Animal species and evolution. Cambridge (MA): Harvard University Press; 1963. p. 162.

9. O'Brien JS, Okada S, Fillerup DL, et al. Tay Sachs disease: prenatal diagnosis. Science 1971;172:61–4.

10. Kaback M, Lim-Steele J, Dabholkar D, et al. Tay-Sachs disease – carrier screening, prenatal diagnosis, and the molecular era. An international perspective, 1970–1993. The International TSD Data Collection Network. JAMA 1993; 270:2307–15.

11. Kaplan F. Tay-Sachs disease carrier screening: a model for prevention of genetic disease. Genet Test 1998;2(4):271–92.

12. Kaback MM. Screening and prevention in Tay-Sachs disease: origins, update, and impact. Adv Genet 2001;44:253–65.

13. Ozelius LJ, Kramer PL, de Leon D, et al. Strong allelic association between the torsion dystonia gene (DYT1) and loci on chromosome 9q34 in Ashkenazi Jews. Am J Hum Genet 1992;50(3):619–28.

14. Leib JR, Gollust SE, Hull SC, et al. Carrier screening panels for Ashkenazi Jews: is more better? Genet Med 2005;7(3):185–90.

15. Gross SJ, Pletcher BA, Monaghan KG. Carrier screening in individuals of Ashkenazi Jewish descent. Genet Med 2008;10(1):54–6.

16. ACOG Committee on Genetics. ACOG Committee Opinion No. 442: preconception and prenatal carrier screening for genetic diseases in individuals of Eastern European Jewish descent. Obstet Gynecol 2009;114:950–3.

17. Pletcher BA, Gross SJ, Monaghan KG, et al. The future is now: carrier screening for all populations. Genet Med 2008;10(1):33–6.

18. Parvari R, Lei K, Bashan N, et al. Glycogen storage disease type 1a in Israel: biochemical, clinical and mutational studies. Am J Med Genet 1998;72:286–90.

19. Edelmann L, Wasserstein MP, Kornreich R, et al. Maple Syrup urine disease: identification and carrier-frequency determination of a novel founder mutation in the Ashkenazi Jewish population. Am J Hum Genet 2001;69(4):863–8.

20. Sansaricq C, Pardo S, Balwani M, et al. Biochemical and molecular diagnosis of lipoamide dehydrogenase deficiency in a North American Ashkenazi Jewish family. J Inherit Metab Dis 2006;29(1):203–4.

21. Nestorowicz A, Wilson BA, Schoor KP, et al. Mutations in the sulfonylurea receptor gene are associated with familial hyperinsulinism in Ashkenazi Jews. Hum Mol Genet 1996;5(11):1813–22.

22. Anderson SL, Ekstein J, Donnelly MC, et al. Nemaline myopathy in the Ashkenazi Jewish population is caused by a deletion in the nebulin gene. Hum Genet 2004; 115(3):185–90.

23. Ben-Yosef T, Ness SL, Madeo AC, et al. A mutation of PCDH15 among Ashkenazi Jews with the type 1 Usher syndrome. N Engl J Med 2003;348(17):1664–70.

24. Ness SL, Ben-Yosef T, Bar-Lev A, et al. Genetic homogeneity and phenotypic variability among Ashkenazi Jews with Usher syndrome type III. J Med Genet 2003;40(10):767–72.

25. ACOG Committee on Genetics. ACOG Committee Opinion. No 318, October 2005. Screening for Tay-Sachs disease. Obstet Gynecol 2005;106(4):893–4.

26. Schneider A, Nakagawa S, Keep R, et al. Population-based Tay-Sachs screening among Ashkenazi Jewish young adults in the 21st century: Hexosaminidase A enzyme assay is essential for accurate testing. Am J Med Genet A 2009; 149(11):2444–7.

27. Bach G, Tomczak J, Risch N, et al. Tay-Sachs screening in the Jewish Ashkenazi population: DNA testing is the preferred procedure. Am J Med Genet 2001;99:70–5.

28. Yoo HW, Astrin KH, Desnick RJ. Comparison of enzyme and DNA analysis in a Tay-Sachs disease carrier screening program. J Korean Med Sci 1993;8:84–91.

29. Available at: http://ntsad.org/events/NTSAD_Position_Statement.pdf. Accessed September 2009.

30. Matalon R, Michals K, Kaul R. Canavan disease: from spongy degeneration to molecular analysis. J Pediatr 1995;127(4):511–7.

31. Kronn D, Oddoux C, Phillips J, et al. Prevalence of Canavan disease I the Ashkenazi Jewish population, implications for counseling and testing. Obstet Gynecol 1995;97:S38–9.

32. Moskowitz SM, Chmiel JF, Sternen DL, et al. Clinical practice and genetic counseling for cystic fibrosis and CFTR-related disorders. Genet Med 2008;10(12): 851–68.

33. Committee on Genetics, American College of Obstetricians and Gynecologists. ACOG Committee Opinion No. 325. Update on carrier screening for cystic fibrosis. Obstet Gynecol 2005;106:1465–8.

34. ACOG Committee on Genetics. ACOG Committee Opinion. No. 298. Prenatal and preconceptional carrier screening for genetic diseases in individuals of Eastern European Jewish descent. Obstet Gynecol 2004;104(2):425–8.

35. Axelrod FB. A world without pain or tears. Clin Auton Res 2006;16(2):90–7.

36. Blumenfeld A, Slaugenhaupt SA, Liebert CB, et al. Precise genetic mapping and haplotype analysis of the familial dysautonomia gene on human chromosome 9q31. Am J Hum Genet 1999;64(4):1110–8.

37. Green AM, Kupfer GM. Fanconi anemia. Hematol Oncol Clin North Am 2009; 23(2):193–214.

38. Schuchman EH, Miranda SR. Niemann-Pick disease: mutation update, genotype/ phenotype correlations, and prospects for genetic testing. Genet Test 1997;1(1): 13–9.

39. Li L, Eng C, Desnick RJ, et al. Carrier frequency of the Bloom syndrome blmAsh mutation in the Ashkenazi Jewish population. Mol Genet Metab 1998;64(4): 286–90.

40. Bach G, Webb MB, Bargal R, et al. The frequency of mucolipidosis type IV in the Ashkenazi Jewish population and the identification of 3 novel MCOLN1 mutations. Hum Mutat 2005;26(6):591.

41. Weinreb NJ, Deegan P, Kacena KA, et al. Life expectancy in Gaucher disease type 1. Am J Hematol 2008;83(12):896–900.

42. Levy-Lahad E, Zuckerman S, Sagi M. Response to ACMG guideline: carrier screening in individuals of Ashkenazi Jewish decent. Genet Med 2008;10(6):462.

Carrier Screening for Cystic Fibrosis

Jeffrey S. Dungan, MD

KEYWORDS

- Cystic fibrosis • Carrier testing • CFTR • Mutation panel

Cystic fibrosis (CF) is an inherited disease with a classic triad of obstructive pulmonary disease, pancreatic insufficiency, and elevated sweat chloride. The appearance of symptoms is typically early in childhood (before age 2 years) with gastrointestinal malabsorption and persistent respiratory complaints as consistent presentations. Exocrine pancreatic insufficiency (PI) is the cause of malabsorption, and occurs as a result of the autodestructive retention of enzymes. PI is present in the majority of infants with CF. About 15% of affected individuals have "pancreatic-sufficient" CF, meaning there is normal or near-normal pancreatic exocrine function, and the long-term prognosis for such individuals is better than for those with classic pancreatic insufficient CF. However, the diagnosis of CF is now made earlier in life with the advent of newborn screening (NBS). As of this writing, all states were either performing NBS for CF, or were scheduled to by the end of 2009. Cystic fibrosis has historically been labeled a lethal disorder, with late childhood deaths the most common outcome. With modern and intensive therapy and surveillance, median life expectancy is now longer than 40 years.[1] Pregnancy in women with cystic fibrosis, while still relatively unusual, is becoming more common than ever before. This article does not deal with the perinatal considerations surrounding pregnancies in affected women, but with the logistics, limitations, and utility of prenatal carrier testing. Carrier testing for CF has become an established part of routine prenatal care in the United States.[2]

DISEASE MANIFESTATIONS

Prior to the advent of routine NBS, most affected children presented as infants, with either gastrointestinal signs/symptoms, pulmonary problems, or both. Approximately 15% of newborns have meconium ileus,[3] which results in bowel obstruction from impacted meconium. Pancreatic insufficiency is manifested by malabsorption sequelae such as greasy stools, abdominal distension, and poor weight gain. Fat-soluble vitamin malabsorption contributes to the malnutrition spectrum. Pharmacologic replacement of pancreatic enzymes controls much of this symptomatology;

Division of Clinical Genetics, Department of Obstetrics & Gynecology, Northwestern University Feinberg School of Medicine, 250 East Superior Street, 05-2168, Chicago, IL 60611, USA
E-mail address: jdungan@nmh.org

Obstet Gynecol Clin N Am 37 (2010) 47–59
doi:10.1016/j.ogc.2010.02.002
0889-8545/10/$ – see front matter
obgyn.theclinics.com

however, vitamin deficiency and overall poor weight gain continue to be significant ongoing medical problems for these patients.

Pulmonary complications appear during early childhood in the form of frequent recurrent coughing and wheezing. Chronic inflammation develops even in the absence of overt infection. Infants may become colonized with *Pseudomonas aeruginosa*, and nearly all children become colonized by 3 years of age.[3] Chronic infection leads ultimately to bronchiectasis and air trapping. Other bacterial species play prominent roles in the pathogenesis of CF lung disease, including *Staphyloccocus aureus* and *Burkholderia cepacia* organisms, all of which are associated with very high rates of antibiotic resistance and extensive tissue damage. Inhaled agents (tobramycin and DNase) are useful in the management of these challenging problems.

Some individuals with CF develop pancreatic endocrine disease as well, although the disease course is different from typical diabetes mellitus. Regular blood glucose screening is part of CF care.

Men with CF are almost always infertile as a result of congenital bilateral absence of the vas deferens (CBAVD). The vas is vulnerable even to the "milder" alleles associated with nonclassic CF (see later discussion). Isolated CBAVD is sometimes considered an atypical, or nonclassic, presentation of CF, and any male with this condition should undergo testing for *CFTR* mutations, even in the absence of respiratory symptoms. A large number of CF mutations are associated with less severe or even absence of the typical disease features. These so-called mild alleles may also result in a disease phenotype that consists of only chronic sinusitis and normal levels of sweat chloride.

The full diagnostic evaluation necessary to establish a diagnosis of CF in nonclassic presentations is beyond the scope of this article, but authoritative sources have reviewed this topic in detail.[4] Measurement of sweat chloride (>60 mEq/L) has long been considered the gold standard for confirmation of CF diagnosis. Diagnostic evaluations as follow-up of positive newborn screens are typically performed by mutation analysis. Sweat chloride testing (also known as quantitative pilocarpine iontophoresis procedure) is also performed in instances of negative mutation analysis to increase diagnostic yield.

MOLECULAR GENETICS AND PATHOPHYSIOLOGY

Cystic fibrosis is almost always caused by alterations or absence of the cystic fibrosis transmembrane conductance regulator (CFTR) protein that spans the cell membrane of most epithelial cells and blood cells. CFTR is a 1480–amino-acid protein with 2 transmembrane domains, 2 nucleotide binding domains (for adenosine triphosphate binding), and an intracellular regulatory domain. Alterations in any of these regions can cause disease manifestations, and the number of identified mutations now exceeds 1500. The *CFTR* gene is found on chromosome 7, consists of 27 exons, and was sequenced in 1989. The most common mutation causing CF is called F508del (previously referred to as delta F508 or ΔF508), so named because of the deletion of the amino acid phenylalanine at position 508 in the protein, a result of a 3-nucleotide deletion in *CFTR* (**Fig. 1**). This mutation results in a folding abnormality of the protein, which ultimately results in protein degradation by normal cellular processes before it even leaves the endoplasmic reticulum.[5]

The physiologic role of CFTR is its action as a chloride channel in the cell membrane. Arrest or inhibition of this ion channel results in absent or reduced efflux of chloride ion from the cell. Although the precise mechanisms by which this disruption results in the phenotypic consequences associated with CF are not completely understood, the end

				deleted			
Normal	Nucleotide	ATC	ATC	TTT	GGT	GTT	
	Amino acid	Ile	Ile	Phe	Gly	Val	
	Position	506	507	508	509	510	
F508del	Nucleotide	ATC	ATT	GGT	GTT		
	Amino acid	Ile	Ile	Gly	Val		

Fig. 1. Sequence of F508del mutation.

results in the respiratory epithelium are reduced water content in secretions, higher salt content, and reduction of water volume in the lumen lined by ciliated epithelium. These secretions become viscous; the small airways are unable to be cleared of mucus, and quickly become colonized with a variety of bacterial pathogens.[3] The concomitant infection and inflammation result in progressive epithelial damage. Thickened mucinous inspissations of the pancreatic ducts are another example of this obstructive progression. With abnormal chloride channel function, there is concomitant impairment of chloride-bicarbonate exchange across the ductal epithelium, and impaired water secretion. This situation results in retention of pancreatic enzymes and progressive tissue damage of pancreatic acini and ducts, leading to cavitation (the "cysts" of cystic fibrosis). A similar process may occur in the hepatic canaliculi as well, resulting in chronic liver damage.

This same ion channel disruption allows for the diagnosis of CF, by measurement of salt content in the sweat of CF patients. Failure of the CFTR to resorb chloride ion from sweat secretions (and in turn, sodium that would normally also be resorbed) results in abnormally high concentrations by the time the sweat fluid reaches the skin surface.[5] The technical aspects of sweat chloride measurement are considerable. In addition, the results may not be abnormal in some cases, making mutation analysis an increasingly more reliable method of diagnosis confirmation.

About half of known *CFTR* mutations are missense (change in amino acid sequence). The remaining mutation types result in premature termination of the amino acid chain, are splice-site mutations, or are frame-shift mutations that alter the reading frame. Commercial testing for carrier detection purposes is designed to screen for the most frequently encountered mutations clinically, and the panel of mutations recommended for routine laboratory screening has been set forth by the American College of Obstetricians and Gynecologists (ACOG) and the American College of Medical Genetics (ACMG). However, when doing clinical testing in individuals suspected of being affected with CF, full gene sequencing may be used, which results in a high overall detection rate.

TYPES OF CFTR MUTATIONS: "SEVERE" VERSUS "MILD" ALLELES

Not all CF mutations result in the traditional form of the disease. With the exception of the 15 to 20 most common known mutations, the bulk of identified mutations are limited to a relatively small number of patients, and have not been well characterized with respect to associated disease phenotype. Mutations have been classified into 5 categories based on the molecular/cellular defect, but the clinical utility of this scheme is unproven and should not be used to predict phenotype.[6] The "milder" forms of CF typically are pancreatic-sufficient (found in <10% of CF patients), and the respiratory issues may be much less extensive. Prior to use of NBS, it was not uncommon for a diagnosis of CF to be made as late as adolescence or early adulthood.[4]

In addition to traditional exonic mutations that result in disease, CFTR function can be altered by certain intronic polymorphisms, the best characterized being the poly-thymidine tract in intron 8 at the exon 9 splice acceptor site (**Fig. 2**). Alterations of normal intron 8 sequence can result in skipping of exon 9 during mRNA transcription, which in turn results in diminished amounts of normal CFTR transcripts. When found in *cis* to the R117H mutation, (ie, is on the same chromosome), the effect can be identical to a "severe" mutation, and thus if this combination exists in conjunction with a classic CFTR mutation, one would predict full manifestations of classic CF. If the R117H mutation exists with the normal 7T (or 9T) allele, the effect is dampened. When *trans* to certain other *CFTR* mutations, the 5T allele can result in mild disease, CBAVD, or sometimes no identifiable disease manifestations.

Routine testing for the poly-T allele is not recommended for carrier identification. Heterozygosity for the 5T allele is fairly common in the general population (5%–7%),[7] and thus many people would unnecessarily be made anxious about this "abnormal" carrier result when, in fact, as an isolated finding it is not expected to result in a child with any CF-related disease (given the partner is not a carrier of any CF mutation). However, it is important to perform poly-T analysis if the R117H mutation is identified, as this combination (in *cis*) is considered a "severe" CF mutation. Likewise, analysis for the 5T allele is performed during the genetic evaluation of males with CBAVD (see later discussion).

EPIDEMIOLOGY

CF is inherited as an autosomal recessive disorder, so carrier parents have a one-quarter, or 25%, chance of an affected child with any pregnancy. Most affected children are born to parents who were unaware of their carrier status. Unaffected sibs of children with CF have a two-thirds chance of being a carrier, making communication with other family members an important part of disease and carrier testing strategies. There is a negligible spontaneous mutation rate in the *CFTR* gene,[4] meaning virtually

Normal sequence (7T allele)

```
        |---7T----|
...gtgtgtgt t t t t t t aacagGGATTT...
                        ↑ intron 8 – exon 9 junction
```

5T allele (results in exon 9 skipping and reduced CFTR mRNA transcript)

```
        |--5T--|
...gtgtgtgt t t t t aacagGGATTT...
```

9T allele (results in normal amount CFTR mRNA transcript)

```
        |----9T------|
...gtgtgtgt t t t t t t t t t aacagGGATTT....
```

Fig. 2. Intron 8 polythymidine tract.

all CF alleles found in affected children have been inherited from obligate carrier parents.

CF is primarily a disease of Caucasians, with a birth incidence of around 1 in 3000. On the other hand, this disorder has been found in virtually all ethnic groups, albeit with variable frequency (**Table 1**). In addition to the disparate prevalence of CF across ethnic groups, the ability to exclude carrier status is also variable. As stated earlier, the number of defined and confirmed mutations in the CFTR gene is greater than1500. The majority of individuals of northern European descent have detectable mutations, with one mutation, F508del (in the homozygous state), being responsible for around three-quarters of CF patients in this population. In other non-Caucasian populations, the proportion of CF patients homozygous for F508del is less than 50%, with many having only one or no identifiable mutation. The 20 most common mutations account for the vast majority of CF alleles worldwide, and after these, no single mutation accounts for more than 0.1% of the total number of mutations detectable in any population. However, several affected individuals from non-Caucasian populations have CF with no or only one detectable mutation.[4]

Reliable detection rates (eg, over 90%) can be easily achieved in homogeneous populations by testing for relatively few mutations, but in more ethnically diverse and mixed areas, a higher number will need to be tested to achieve such high detection rates. For example, in France over 300 mutations need to be screened to achieve comparable detection rates.[4] Likewise, in a series of Hispanic CF patients residing in California, the percentage of mutations detected was 65% using basic screening panels such as that endorsed by the ACMG. Expanded molecular analysis using sophisticated mutation detection techniques can raise the detection rate to 94.5%, identifying several rare and novel mutations.[8] This fact is tempered by the lower incidence of affected CF patients in this ethnic group, and the ideal approach to carrier screening under such conditions is undetermined. Some of the mutations found in this group of Hispanic patients have been added to the commercially available expanded mutation panels.

Expanded knowledge of the mutations associated with CF has not resulted in an ability to predict genotype-phenotype correlation, particularly with respect to lung disease. The most common homozygous F508del genotype is associated with the typical full CF clinical picture, but even in these individuals the course of pulmonary disease is unpredictable and variable across patients with the same CF genotype,

Table 1		
Incidence of cystic fibrosis in various populations		
Ethnic Group	**Disease Incidence**	**Carrier Frequency**
Caucasian	1/3200	1/28
Ashkenazi Jewish	1/3300	1/29
African American	1/17000	1/65
Asian American	1/25500	1/80
Hispanic	1/11500	1/53
Native American[a]	1/10500	1/50

[a] Higher frequencies found in certain Native American populations; for example, amongst Zunis, incidence is 1/1580.

Data from American Lung Association Web site. Research-data & statistics—State of Lung Disease in Diverse Communities – lung disease data at a glance: cystic fibrosis – racial/ethnic differences. Available at: http://www.lungusa.org. Accessed November 10, 2009.

including within a sibship. Although a series of genetic modifiers has been investigated,[9] use of this information to predict phenotype is not appropriate for genetic counseling purposes. The extent to which environmental factors influence disease course is also of prime importance, but difficult to quantify. Further research may uncover consistent polymorphisms in other genes, such as TGFβ1, which impact disease phenotype, but for now this remains investigational.

CLINICAL ASPECTS OF CARRIER TESTING

Carrier testing is typically performed early in prenatal care, but is ideally performed preconceptionally, so that carrier parents may explore all of their reproductive options. However, apparently very few obstetricians are discussing or offering this testing to preconceptional patients.[2] When carrier testing reveals CFTR mutations in both parents, testing options for the fetus are limited to invasive procedures (chorionic villus sampling [CVS], amniocentesis) with the option for termination of an affected fetus. Preconceptional knowledge of carrier status allows for other options, such as preimplantation genetic diagnosis (PGD) or gamete donation. Successful pregnancies have resulted from PGD cycles to exclude affected embryos from transfer, the first such live birth being reported in 1992.[10]

Preconceptionally, at-risk couples should be told of options: PGD, donor gametes, and invasive prenatal testing. In early pregnancy, they should undergo genetic counseling and discussion of invasive testing. Most couples who learn of an affected fetus decide to terminate those pregnancies.[11,12] The number of at-risk couples (as determined by identification of affected child through clinical or NBS methods) who decline invasive testing in subsequent pregnancies is reported to range from 33% to 80%.[12] The proportion of at-risk couples who choose to undergo PGD versus natural conception followed by invasive prenatal genetic testing is unknown, but is likely not a high proportion of known at-risk couples given the necessity and expense of the in vitro fertilization interventions.

Both ACOG and ACMG recommend use of a 23-mutation panel as the preferred approach to mutation testing (**Table 2**). With these 23 most common mutations, the majority of carriers will be identified (**Table 3**), at least in those populations with highest carrier frequency.[13] For low-risk patients, as a matter of universal screening, this approach is sufficient. One can see by comparing **Tables 1** and **3** that with decreased prevalence in a given population, the detection rate likewise diminishes. Such information is vital to provide accurate risk counseling to patients. However, in instances of a positive family history of affected individuals, but with no known mutation, further

Table 2 Mutation panel recommended by ACOG and ACMG (listed in order of decreasing frequency in non-Hispanic Caucasian population)			
F508 del	delI507	R347P	R1162X
G542X	R553X	711+1G>T	2184delA
G551D	R117H	R560T	1898+1G>A
621+1G>T	3849+10kbC>T	3569delC	R334W
W1282X	1717−1G>T	A455E	3120+1G>T
N1303K	2789+5G>A	G85E	

Data from Watson MS, Cutting GR, Desnick RJ, et al. Cystic fibrosis population carrier screening: 2004 revision of American College of Medical Genetics mutation panel. Genet Med 2004;6:387–91.

Table 3	
Detection rate of CF carriers with use of 23-mutation panel as recommended by ACOG and ACMG	
Ethnicity	**Detection Rate of CF Mutations by 23-Mutation Panel (%)**
Ashkenazi Jewish	94.0
Caucasian	88.3
Hispanic	71.9
African American	64.5
Asian American	48.9
Combined ethnicities	83.9

Data from Watson MS, Cutting GR, Desnick RJ, et al. Cystic fibrosis population carrier screening: 2004 revision of American College of Medical Genetics mutation panel. Genet Med 2004;6:387–91.

evaluation of the patient's mutation status by means of expanded mutation panels or gene sequencing may be appropriate (assuming of course the first-tier 23-mutation panel was negative).

Although a variety of approaches for carrier testing exist (eg, both members of the couple simultaneously), for practical reasons, testing of the pregnant (or preconceptional) female initially is the most widespread practice. When she is identified as a carrier, the partner should undergo carrier testing. In the absence of a paternal family history of CF, the standard mutation panel is considered sufficient for testing of this partner. If a Caucasian patient is found to have a positive mutation screen, but her partner's testing is negative, the risk of this couple having an affected infant is calculated as such:

1/2 (risk of known carrier to transmit CF allele) × 1/208 (risk partner is still carrier after negative mutation testing) × 1/2 (risk of transmitting that unknown allele) = 1/832

By means of Bayesian analysis, more accurate risk calculations in a variety of other circumstances, including ethnic differences, can be made to determine an individual's risk to be a carrier. The example in **Box 1** illustrates how this information can be used. Such calculations are performed routinely in the clinical setting to help patients decide about further testing.

A review of the Bayesian analysis techniques used in counseling patients with positive family histories, unknown mutation status, or other mitigating circumstances can be found elsewhere.[14,15] Geneticists and genetic counselors will be able to provide the most accurate risk counseling in complex scenarios.

The ACMG guidelines on CF carrier testing state that intron 8 poly-T analysis should be reported only as a reflex if the R117H allele is found (see section on "severe" versus "mild" alleles). Despite the lack of predictable or consistent phenotype associated with the 5T intron 8 allele in conjunction with any mutation other than R117H, a considerable number of laboratories performing carrier testing for CF in the United States still report the 5T allele on all specimens.[16] This activity has led to unnecessary invasive prenatal testing whereby parents are not at risk of having a child with CF, and misunderstand the significance (or lack thereof) of the 5T allele.[17,18] While such situations are generally rare, these events reflect the complexity of carrier testing strategies for this particular disorder, and the continued need for provider education.

> **Box 1**
> **Bayesian analysis to calculate risk of being carrier of CF mutation**
>
> Bayesian analysis calculates chances of 2 scenarios: being a carrier or NOT being a carrier, depending on the various parameters set up by the presentation. Assume that the 23-mutation panel detects 88% of the CF mutations in her ethnic group.
>
> AB is a Caucasian nulliparous woman who presents for prenatal CF risk assessment. Her deceased father had a sister who died of cystic fibrosis as a child, and no mutation testing was available at the time. Your patient, AB, underwent routine carrier testing that was negative for the 23 mutations on the panel. What is her residual risk for being a carrier of a *CFTR* mutation?
>
> | | AB is a Carrier | AB is NOT a Carrier |
> | --- | --- | --- |
> | Prior probability (based on the fact her father had 2/3 chance of being a carrier) | 1/3 (0.33) | 2/3 (0.67) |
> | Conditional probability (based on her negative mutation testing) | 0.12 (1–0.88) | 1 |
> | Joint probability (product of prior × conditional) | 0.04 | 0.667 |
> | Posterior probability (joint/sum of both joint probabilities) | 0.057 | 0.943 |
>
> Thus, your patient AB has an approximately 5% to 6% chance of being a carrier of an undetected CFTR mutation, which may be an indication for extended panel testing or gene sequencing if she requested further risk assessment.

The general practice obstetrician-gynecologist should be able to facilitate carrier testing in uncomplicated cases. Referral to a genetic or maternal-fetal medicine specialist is appropriate when:

- A couple has a previous child with CF
- One or both partners is found to be carriers of a CF mutation
- One or both partners has a positive family history of CF or CBAVD
- Patients have questions about CF or carrier testing in general that are outside the domain of her regular obstetric care provider.

EXPANDED MUTATION SCREENING/FULL GENE SEQUENCING

Several laboratories offer mutation testing more extensive than that recommended by ACMG or ACOG.[19] The additional usefulness of such options is uncertain. In populations with high detection rates achievable with traditional means (eg, Ashkenazi Jewish), these more extensive and costly testing options certainly offer no discernible benefit. Where these expanded panels may have clinically useful roles is in the screening/testing of individuals from populations with low carrier detection rates, such as Asian Americans, especially in cases with a positive family history. The benefit of expanded testing even in this scenario, however, is open to debate.

In a Commentary article, Grody and colleagues[20] criticize the "arms race" mentality of laboratories offering larger and larger mutation panels. There are no data supporting the enhanced detection of carriers, nor is there information on expected phenotype of individuals in whom 1 or 2 of these rarer mutations exist. Current technology does not even allow for facile determination of whether 2 mutations are on the same or opposite chromosomes (this would require extended family studies). Indeed, these investigators cite studies demonstrating considerable added expense in routinely using expanded panels versus the recommended "core" panel, with *no* increased diagnostic yield from more than 500 patient samples. From other studies, only those individuals from families with positive CF histories were ever found to have any of the mutations not routinely detected by the core panel, and this added detection rate was only 6 out of 167 (3.6%). Full gene sequencing is certainly associated with high detection rates of mutation regardless of patient ethnicity. However, the likelihood of detecting variants of uncertain clinical significance likewise is increased. Evidence-based counseling in such circumstances is virtually impossible. This fact, along with the considerably higher cost of such testing, should dissuade the clinician from pursuing this line of testing for routine purposes.

HISTORY OF PRENATAL CARRIER TESTING FOR CF

Years of debate preceded the introduction of CF carrier testing as routine and standard part of prenatal care. Many of the objections were initiated because of the complexity of *CFTR* mutations, and the need for widespread education of medical professionals not accustomed to dealing with genetic disorders. While screening for carriers of other single gene disorders had been in place for years (eg, Tay-Sachs), the disease phenotype of those disorders was more well-defined, and the populations eligible for testing were somewhat more distinct. CF is the first genetic disorder for which universal carrier testing was introduced into common clinical practice.

Finally, in 2001 a joint statement was made by ACOG and ACMG[21] that stated, in addition to offering testing to patients with a positive family history of CF, all patients of Caucasian or Ashkenazi Jewish descent should be offered carrier screening. A core 25-mutation panel was recommended at the same time to guide laboratories that performed such testing. Because of the ethnic differences in carrier prevalence, these guidelines differentiated the type of clinical approach that should be taken based on ethnic background. For populations with the highest carrier frequency (ie, Northern European descendants, Ashkenazi Jewish descendants), the care provider was instructed to discuss the availability of carrier testing and to offer such testing. For other ethnic groups, merely making this testing "available" (defined as written material that could be handed out vs spending time discussing with the patient) was considered appropriate. Although the recommended mutation panel has subsequently been changed slightly,[13] the mandates to obstetric care providers remains the same. Carrier testing for CF should be offered to all Caucasian, Ashkenazi Jewish, or European patients seeking prenatal or preconceptional care.[2] Information on CF and carrier testing should be available to all patients, regardless of ethnicity. Because some practitioners find it confusing to differentiate these 2 categories of carrier testing approaches, and identification of single or uniform ethnicity is less readily available, the guidelines were updated in 2005. These guidelines now state that it is reasonable to undertake a policy of offering testing to all prenatal or preconceptional patients, regardless of ethnic background.[2] On the other hand, neither universal nor ethnic-based CF carrier testing is performed in all countries (eg, Canada). The Society of Obstetricians and Gynaecologists of Canada has stated routine CF carrier screening "cannot be recommended at this time."[22]

Two mutations were subsequently deleted from the original 2001 recommendation as a result of further epidemiologic data.[13] The I148T mutation was subsequently found *not* to be disease causing (it was originally considered so because of the erroneous perception of its frequent appearance with 3199del6, a rare, but confirmed CF mutation). The other mutation (1078delT) was removed because of its rarity.

MALE INFERTILITY AND CFTR MUTATIONS

Azoospermia is a common explanation for male infertility. One cause of obstructive azoospermia is CBAVD, a condition found in nearly all males with a clinical diagnosis of CF. One to two percent of infertile men have CBAVD. Chillon and colleagues[23] analyzed a series of men with either unilateral or bilateral absence of the vas deferens (ie, not previously identified as having CF), and found about 19% had 2 identified mutations and 72% had at least one identifiable mutation, including the 5T allele in intron 8. On the other hand, infertile males with nonobstructive azoospermia, or who have other causes of infertility, have not been found to have a higher likelihood of being a CF carrier than the general population.[24] Thus, males presenting with CBAVD should undergo CFTR mutation analysis as part of their diagnostic evaluation, as well as before initiation of sperm retrieval interventions. Likewise, their female partners should undergo carrier screening. Unless the male with CBAVD undergoes expanded CFTR mutation analysis or full CFTR sequencing, there will remain some residual risk of carrying an unidentified CFTR mutation (depending on mutation panel used). Knowledge of the prospective mother's carrier status will allow more accurate risk assessment in this complex scenario. Most couples with this presentation benefit from formal genetic counseling.

INVASIVE PRENATAL TESTING FOR AT-RISK PREGNANCIES

When both members of a couple have identified CF mutations, prenatal testing in the form of CVS or amniocentesis must be offered. In current practice, all prenatal CF diagnoses are made by mutation analysis. Prior to mutation testing of *CFTR*, measurement of microvillar enzymes in the amniotic fluid had been used to predict affected fetuses, but these assays suffer from overall poor specificity and now are of historical interest only.

In about 1% of routine fetal anatomy sonograms, the bowel will appear echogenic. This finding has been associated with increased risk of a fetus affected with CF. Full perspective on this finding has been discussed in detail.[25] Overall, the risk for fetal CF is reported to be around 1% to 3%, depending on disease prevalence in the specific population. By contrast, a minority of fetuses affected with CF actually demonstrate echogenic bowel in the second trimester. A great deal of parental anxiety can be allayed by knowledge of their carrier status before the sonogram takes place. If a sonogram demonstrates echogenic bowel, and parental carrier status has not previously been determined, parental carrier testing should be offered. Because this sonographic finding has also been associated with increased fetal aneuploidy risk, the patient may decide to proceed with amniocentesis before any knowledge of her and her partner's CF carrier status. In these situations, laboratories will typically hold cultured fetal cells for *CFTR* testing, pending completion of the parental testing. No fetal testing is performed if mutations are not identified in the parents. Because of the incomplete mutation detectability, the couple will need to be made aware of their reduced, but not eliminated, risk of an affected child.

PATIENT ACCEPTANCE/UPTAKE OF CARRIER TESTING

Researchers have examined patient uptake and preferences surrounding carrier testing for CF. Not surprisingly, there is wide variability across demographic groups with respect to request for carrier testing.[26] In a systematic review of studies examining patient preferences regarding carrier testing, Chen and Goodson[26] reported summary averages of 48% of preconceptional patient testing uptake, and around 74% in the prenatal setting. As previously stated, research also confirms that the majority of at-risk couples who pursue prenatal diagnosis decide to terminate those pregnancies found to be affected.

In this systematic review, certain factors were consistently shown to be associated with the decision to accept or decline testing:

Factors Leading to Acceptance of CF Carrier Testing	Factors Associated With Declining CF Carrier Testing
Personal benefit of knowing carrier status (can prevent birth of affected child)	Perceived "barriers" to testing, eg, cost, fear of blood draw
No previous children	Multiparity
Desire to assist with research	Lack of knowledge about CF
Higher socioeconomic status	Antiabortion stance
Caucasian race	

In an informative Australian study reported by Sawyer and colleagues,[12] parents of children with CF who had been detected by NBS were not only generally supportive of prenatal CF testing (82% stated they would pursue prenatal testing in any subsequent pregnancy), but slightly more than half stated they would terminate another pregnancy if the fetus was found to be affected. This same cohort was then resurveyed 5 years later, specifically addressing actual reproductive outcomes. About 60% of the mothers of children with CF went on to have subsequent pregnancies, and in two out of 3 of these pregnancies, prenatal diagnosis for CF was performed. In the small cohort (5/33) of affected pregnancies, all were terminated, consistent with other studies examining this question.[11] Eighty-nine percent of the mothers whose prenatal testing excluded CF stated they would have terminated the pregnancy if testing had demonstrated an affected fetus. Also quite telling was that women's decisions and attitudes about prenatal testing changed in both directions between the original survey and the follow-up 5 years later. Prenatal care providers should be reoffering carrier testing to women/couples in subsequent pregnancies even if it had previously been declined.

IMPACT OF CARRIER TESTING ON BIRTH INCIDENCE OF CF

One measure of the effectiveness of a screening program is determining whether the birth incidence of the disorder in question is altered (decreased); this would reflect an impact on reproductive outcomes (avoidance of pregnancy, termination of affected pregnancies) in those couples identified as being at risk. Another potential source of reduction in birth incidence would be carrier parents' use of alternative reproductive technologies (ie, preimplantation genetic diagnoses, donor gametes) to achieve pregnancy, although this latter option would not likely account for a large effect.

Hale and colleagues[27] report that since 2001, the birth incidence of CF in Massachusetts has declined from 25 to 30 infants per year to around 15 per year in 2005 and 2006. The relative proportion of F508del homozygous newborns has also declined substantially, indicating the impact of carrier identification and avoidance of affected newborns by means of prenatal testing or avoidance of pregnancy in at-risk couples.

A similar phenomenon was reported from Italy,[28] where carrier screening has been available in the eastern region of the country for several years. A significant reduction in birth incidence was noted (all diagnoses made through NBS) from 1993 to 2007. During this interval, there was an annual reduction of 0.24 per 10,000, from about 4 per 10,000 birth incidence at the beginning of carrier testing to about 1.5 per 10,000 newborns affected at the end of the study interval. Of note, in the western region of the country, which otherwise carries a similar population ethnically, there is no widespread implementation of carrier testing and there was a negligible reduction in birth incidence in that part of the country during the study interval.

SUMMARY

Prenatal carrier screening for cystic fibrosis is a routine part of prenatal care. The practicing obstetrician should be familiar with basic aspects of the disease and the limitations of carrier testing. Most patients who opt to undergo such testing will receive reassuring news. In instances where both parents are carriers, referral for prenatal testing should be undertaken without delay. While not perfect, carrier testing is associated overall with a level of accuracy high enough to warrant population screening. With improved treatment regimens and the widespread implementation of NBS, it remains to be seen whether prenatal carrier testing for CF will continue to be accepted at current levels by patients.

REFERENCES

1. Boucher RC. Chapter 253. Cystic fibrosis. In: Fauci AS, Braunwald E, Kasper DL, et al, editors. Harrison's principles of internal medicine. 17th edition. New York: McGraw-Hill; 2008. p. 1632–5.
2. American College of Obstetricians and Gynecologists Committee. Update on carrier screening for cystic fibrosis. Opinion #325. Obstet Gynecol 2005;106(6): 1465–8.
3. O'Sullivan BP, Freedman SD. Cystic fibrosis. Lancet 2009;373:1891–904.
4. Cutting GR. Cystic fibrosis. In: Rimoin DL, Connor JM, Pyeritz RE, et al, editors. Emery and Rimoin's principles and practice of medical genetics. 5th edition. Philadelphia: Churchill Livingstone Elsevier; 2007. p. 1354–79, Chapter 62.
5. Rowe SM, Miller S, Sorscher EJ. Mechanisms of disease: cystic fibrosis. N Engl J Med 2005;352:1992–2001.
6. Castellani C, Cuppens H, Macek M Jr, et al. Consensus on the use and interpretation of cystic fibrosis mutation analysis in clinical practice. J Cyst Fibros 2008;7: 179–96.
7. Kiesewetter S, Macek M Jr, Davis C, et al. A mutation in CFTR produces different phenotypes depending on chromosomal background. Nat Genet 1993;5:274–8.
8. Alper OM, Wong L-J, Young S, et al. Identification of novel and rare mutations in California Hispanics and African American cystic fibrosis patients. Hum Mutat 2004;24:353–67.
9. Drumm ML, Konstan MW, Schluchter MD, et al. Genetic modifiers of lung disease in cystic fibrosis. N Engl J Med 2005;353:1443–53.
10. Handyside AH, Lesko JG, Tarin JJ, et al. Birth of a normal girl after in vitro fertilization and preimplantation diagnostic testing for cystic fibrosis. N Engl J Med 1992;327:905–9.
11. Scotet V, de Braekeleer M, Roussey M, et al. Neonatal screening for cystic fibrosis in Brittany, France: assessment of 10 years experience and impact on prenatal diagnosis. Lancet 2000;356:789–94.

12. Sawyer SM, Cerritelli B, Carter LS, et al. Changing their minds with time: a comparison of hypothetical and actual reproductive behaviors in parents of children with cystic fibrosis. Pediatrics 2006;118:e649–56.
13. Watson MS, Cutting GR, Desnick RJ, et al. Cystic fibrosis population carrier screening: 2004 revision of American College of Medical Genetics mutation panel [published errata appear in Genet Med 2004;6:548; Genet Med 2005;7:286]. Genet Med 2004;6:387–91.
14. Lebo RV, Grody WW. Testing and reporting ACMG cystic fibrosis mutation panel results. Genet Test 2007;11:11–31.
15. Ogino S, Wilson RB, Gold B, et al. Bayesian analysis for cystic fibrosis risks in prenatal and carrier screening. Genet Med 2004;6:439–49.
16. Kaufman DJ, Katsanis SH, Javitt GH, et al. Carrier screening for cystic fibrosis in US genetic testing laboratories: a survey of laboratory directors. Clin Genet 2008; 74:367–73.
17. Rohlfs EM, Weinblatt VJ, Treat KJ, et al. Analysis of 3208 cystic fibrosis prenatal diagnoses: impact of carrier screening guidelines on distribution of indications for CFTR mutation and IVS-8 poly(T) analyses. Genet Med 2004;6:400–4.
18. Vastag B. Cystic fibrosis gene testing a challenge. JAMA 2003;289:2923–4.
19. GeneTests: medical genetics information resource. University of Washington, Seattle. 1993–2010. Available at: http://www.genetests.org. Accessed November 19, 2009.
20. Grody WW, Cutting GR, Watson MS. The cystic fibrosis mutation "arms race": when less is more. Genet Med 2007;9:739–44.
21. American College of Obstetricians and Gynecologists and American College of Medical Genetics. Preconception and prenatal carrier screening for cystic fibrosis. Clinical and laboratory guidelines. Washington, DC: American College of Obstetricians and Gynecologists; 2001.
22. Genetics and Maternal Fetal Medicine Committees of the Society of Obstetricians and Gynaecologists of Canada. Cystic fibrosis carrier testing in pregnancy in Canada. SOGC Committee Opinion No. 118. J Obstet Gynaecol Can 2002;24: 644–7.
23. Chillon M, Casals T, Mercier B, et al. Mutations in the cystic fibrosis gene in patients with congenital absence of the vas deferens. N Engl J Med 1995;332: 1475–80.
24. Mak V, Zielenski J, Tsui L-C, et al. Proportion of cystic fibrosis gene mutations not detected by routine testing in men with obstructive azoospermia. JAMA 1999; 281:2217–24.
25. Slotnick RN, Abuhamad A. Prognostic implications of fetal echogenic bowel. Lancet 1996;347:85–7.
26. Chen L-S, Goodson P. Factors affecting decisions to accept or decline cystic fibrosis carrier testing/screening: a theory-guided systematic review. Genet Med 2007;9:442–50.
27. Hale JE, Parad RB, Comeau AM. Newborn screening showing decreasing incidence of cystic fibrosis [letter]. N Engl J Med 2008;358:973–4.
28. Castellani C, Picci L, Tamanini A, et al. Association between carrier screening and incidence of cystic fibrosis. JAMA 2009;302:2573–9.

Prenatal Carrier Testing for Fragile X: Counseling Issues and Challenges

Thomas J. Musci, MD[a,*], Krista Moyer, MGC[a,b]

KEYWORDS

- Fragile X • Prenatal carrier testing • Prenatal counseling
- Population screening

Mutations of the FMR1 gene (or fragile X mental retardation protein) can affect both the reproductive health of women and cause developmental disabilities in their offspring. The most well-known FMR1-associated disorder is "fragile X syndrome" (FXS), the most common cause of inherited mental impairment and autism or autistic-like behavior. Healthy women who carry a "premutation" in the FMR1 gene can pass on a further mutated copy of FMR1 to either male or female offspring, leading to FXS. Because the FMR1 gene resides on the X chromosome, males are affected more profoundly than females, leading to disease incidence figures in the range of 1 in 3600 for males and 1 in 4000 to 6000 for females (National Fragile X Foundation; http://www.fragilex.org). The frequency of FMR1 premutation allele carriers in the general population is not precisely known; however, recent United States data indicate a carrier frequency of 1 in 86, for those with a family history of mental retardation and 1 in 257 for women with no known risk factors for FXS.[1] A large Israeli study of greater than 36,000 low-risk women indicated a carrier frequency of 1 in 157.[2]

FRAGILE X–ASSOCIATED DISORDERS

Although premutation carriers do not have manifestations of FXS in cognitive deficits, behavioral abnormalities, or classic physical features, they are at increased risk for development of the "fragile X–associated disorders": premature ovarian failure and fragile X–associated tremor and ataxia syndrome.[3,4]

[a] San Francisco Perinatal Associates, Inc, One Daniel Burnham Court, Suite 230 C, San Francisco, CA 94109, USA
[b] Clinical Laboratories, University of California San Francisco Medical Center, 185 Berry Street, Suite 290, San Francisco, CA 94107, USA
* Corresponding author.
E-mail address: tmusci@sfperinatal.com

Obstet Gynecol Clin N Am 37 (2010) 61–70
doi:10.1016/j.ogc.2010.03.004
0889-8545/10/$ – see front matter © 2010 Elsevier Inc. All rights reserved.

Of prime concern during the reproductive years is premature ovarian failure or what is now commonly referred to as fragile X–associated primary ovarian insufficiency (FXPOI).[5] FXPOI, a decline of ovarian function leading to menopause by age 40, can be seen in approximately 20% of women who carry a premutation, compared with 1% of women in the general population.[6,7] In the past few years there has been the suggestion that even women with intermediate zone CGG repeats may be at some risk for ovarian dysfunction and infertility,[8] with varying cut-offs for intermediate sizes reported.[9,10] However, the largest study completed to date did not demonstrate a relationship between intermediate size CGG repeats and the incidence of premature ovarian failure and concluded that these alleles should not be considered a high-risk factor for POF based on current evidence.[11] It should be noted that although this ovarian dysfunction has significant reproductive implications, it does not eliminate the possibility of subsequent spontaneous conceptions. Women identified as carriers of a premutation allele should be counseled as to the risk of ovarian dysfunction, the reproductive implications, and the reproductive options (adoption, assisted reproductive technologies, ovum donation, preimplantation genetic diagnosis, and so forth.) that are available to them. Thus, screening women in their early reproductive years for a possible genetic predisposition to a higher rate of reproductive failure might allow them to monitor their ovarian function early enough to better achieve their reproductive goals.

Fragile X–associated tremor/ataxia syndrome (FXTAS) is a neurodegenerative disorder associated with a late onset (>50 years). Both male and female premutation carriers are at increased risk of developing FXTAS.[12] The disorder consists of intention tremor, ataxia, parkinsonism, neuropathy, specific magnetic resonance imaging findings, and cognitive decline.[4,13] The penetrance of FXTAS is age dependent, with an approximate risk of 40% among male carriers older than 50 years,[14] and 8% in female carriers older than 40 years.[15]

FRAGILE X GENETICS

Whereas the FMR1 gene is located on the X chromosome and can be thought of in classic terms of X-linked disease, the molecular mechanisms of mutations leading to phenotypic manifestations is indeed complex. FXS is caused by expansion of a repeated trinucleotide segment of DNA (a so-called trinucleotide repeat disorder) in the 5-prime untranslated region of the gene (nucleotides: cytosine-guanine-guanine [CGG]), that leads to altered transcription of the fragile X mental retardation 1 (FMR1) gene. The number of CGG repeats varies among individuals and has been classified into 4 groups (**Table 1**): unaffected (<45 repeats), intermediate (45–54 repeats), premutation (55–200 repeats), and full mutation (>200 repeats).[16] When more than 200 repeats are present, an individual is considered to have a full mutation that results in the full expression of FXS in males and variable expression in females. The repeat size in a full mutation allele causes the FMR1 gene to become methylated and transcriptionally silent, with little to no FMR1 protein production. The standard molecular techniques of Southern blot analysis and polymerase chain reaction (PCR) are used to determine both the repeat size and the status of gene methylation.

EXPANSION OF THE FMR1 TRIPLET REPEAT

Transmission of a disease-producing mutation to a fetus can occur only through the female parent and the risk of expansion of the FMR1 gene to a full mutation in the fetus increases with the number of CGG repeats present in the maternal gene (**Table 2**).[17] This instability of the FMR1 gene, and thus expansion of the repeat region to a full

Table 1
Types of fragile X mutations

Mutation Type	Number of CGG Repeats
Unaffected	<45
Intermediate	45–54
Premutation	55–200
Full mutation	>200

Adapted from Kronquist KE, Sherman SL, Spector EB. Clinical significance of tri-nucleotide repeats in fragile X testing: a clarification of American College of Medical Genetics guidelines. Genet Med 2008;10(11):845–7.

mutation, is a key feature of the molecular disease mechanism. The gene characteristics and mechanisms that lead to repeat instability is an area of intense research interest, and are not currently well understood.[18,19]

Women who carry a premutation can transmit either their normal or premutation allele, which may expand, resulting in the birth of an affected child. The smallest repeat size that was previously reported to expand to a full mutation in one generation is 59 repeats.[17] However, a recent report of a single-generation expansion to a full mutation allele (male with approximately 538 CCG repeats) from a mother carrying a premutation allele of 56 CGG repeats underscores the gaps in knowledge surrounding the mechanisms leading to repeat instability. Because in that case report the maternal grandfather was a carrier of an intermediate-zone allele of 52 CGG repeats, it is a unique example of an intermediate allele expanding to a full mutation range in 2 generations.[20] A male premutation carrier will transmit the unexpanded premutation gene to all of his daughters and none of his sons, and is therefore considered at negligible risk of having a child with FXS.

RNA-MEDIATED PATHOGENESIS OF FRAGILE X–ASSOCIATED DISORDERS

In contrast to transcriptional silencing of the FMR1 gene and loss of FMR1 protein in FXS, entirely different molecular mechanisms seem to underlie the fragile X–associated disorders of FXPOI and FXTAS. There is ample evidence now that carriers of

Table 2
Risks of expansion based on number of triplet repeats

Maternal CGG Repeat Size	Total Maternal Transmissions	% Expanded to Full Mutations
55–59	27	3.7
60–69	113	5.3
70–79	90	31.1
80-89	140	57.8
90–99	111	80.1
100–109	70	100
110–119	54	98.1
120–129	36	97.2
130–139	18	94.4
140–200	19	100

Adapted from Nolin SL, Brown WT, Glicksman A, et al. Expansion of the fragile X CGG repeat in females with premutation or intermediate alleles. Am J Hum Genet 2003;72(2):454–64.

Table 3	
Odds ratio for POI based on number of triplet repeats	
Number of CGG Repeats	**Odds Ratio for POI**
59–79	6.9
80–99	25.1
>100	16.4

Adapted from Sullivan AK, Marcus M, Epstein MP, et al. Association of FMR1 repeat size with ovarian dysfunction. Hum Reprod 2005;20:402–12.

premutation alleles (55–200 CGG repeats) of the FMR1 gene have significantly elevated levels of FMR1 mRNA compared with individuals with normal repeat lengths as measured in peripheral blood leukocytes and central nervous system tissue.[21] This increase in cellular FMR1 mRNA is the result of increased transcription.

Whether or not in the case of FXPOI increased levels of FMR1 mRNA play a direct role in the pathogenesis of ovarian dysfunction, it seems clear that the penetrance, age of onset of FXPOI, and increase in follicle-stimulating hormone levels correlate with (CGG) repeat length (**Table 3**).[22] However, there appears to be a nonlinear relationship between the age of onset and the premutation CGG repeat size. Premutations that are considered in the mid-range (approximately 80–99 repeats) apparently confer the greatest risk for premature ovarian failure.[6] In addition, there is further evidence suggesting that additional genetic factors may play a role in the overall risk of premature menopause, as seen in familial aggregation of age of menopause.[3]

In contrast to FXPOI, there has been some recent progress in the elucidation of the underlying mechanisms of the FXTAS. Studies have demonstrated that penetrance increases with both age and CGG repeat length. The incidence of disease is at least 50% in men aged 70–90 years (**Table 4**).[14] The working hypothesis that has gained considerable attention is a model whereby the increased levels of FMRP1 mRNA, seen in premutation carriers, is toxic to neurons and associated with FMR1 RNA-rich intranuclear inclusions and ultimately neurodegeneration.[23] This model is referred to as the "RNA toxic gain-of-function," and evidence gathered from both cell and animal models has provided significant scientific support for the plausibility of this model.

FRAGILE X CARRIER SCREENING

Despite recent interest in widespread carrier screening for FMR1 mutations in the prenatal setting, current consensus guidelines from multiple professional organizations (American Congress of Obstetricians and Gynecologists, American College of

Table 4	
Risk of FXTAS in male premutation carriers based on age	
Age in Years	**Risk in %**
50–59	17
60–69	38
70–79	47
≥80	75

Adapted from Jacquemont S, Hagerman RJ, Leehey MA, et al. Penetrance of the fragile X-associated tremor/ataxia syndrome in a premutation carrier population. JAMA 2004;291:460–9.

Medical Genetics, National Society of Genetic Counselors) have not recommended universal carrier testing. Carrier testing is recommended for those women with a family history of FXS, for those women with ovarian insufficiency, and for those women with a family history of undiagnosed mental retardation, developmental delay, or autism. Testing for premutations is also recommended in men and women with late-onset intention tremor and cerebellar ataxia, especially those individuals with a family history of FXS, unknown mental retardation, and movement disorders.[5,24,25] However, there appears to be growing interest in more liberal screening for fragile X among certain educated patient groups and among medical professionals. Indeed, commercial laboratories have begun marketing fragile X carrier testing to prenatal patients through education pamphlets supplied to obstetric and prenatal diagnosis clinics and offices.[26,27]

An important feature in the consideration of fragile X screening with regard to fragile X carriers, although not unique to this gene, is that the premutation carrier status is silent with regard to a given individual's awareness of their risk for delivering an affected child. It is clear that using only risk-based screening protocols will not detect the majority of premutation carriers in the population,[28] but it does indeed target a higher prevalence group with regard to carrier frequency.

When considering any widespread screening programs in a prenatal setting, several general principles of disease screening are usually applied.[29-31] Foremost, the disease must be clinically significant, with a severity such that prenatal detection is warranted. Options must be available for at-risk individuals, including accurate diagnostic options for fetal testing and choice regarding continuation of a pregnancy. In the case of FXS, particularly in male fetuses as noted, the severity of the phenotype might appropriately prompt invasive fetal testing in a pregnant patient who is a carrier. In addition, the screening test should be inexpensive, with an adequate sensitivity and specificity. There are many features of fragile X that appear to fulfill much of the criteria considered for widespread screening, but discussions regarding costs have had limited attention.

MOLECULAR TESTING: SCREENING VERSUS DIAGNOSTIC ASSAYS

Cost-effectiveness analyses that have been published on fragile X carrier screening demonstrate that for widespread screening protocols to succeed and become adopted, significant cost reduction in fragile X mutation analysis assays will be necessary.[32] Diagnostic FMR1 mutation analysis (number of repeats are precisely determined) currently involves both a PCR and a Southern blot assay, which combined are costly and labor intensive, have prolonged turnaround times, and ultimately have limited utility for population-based screening. The development of lower-cost assays intended for screening (as opposed to current diagnostic assays) will necessitate a change in thinking away from using expensive diagnostic tests toward the use of methods that reliably detect a triplet repeat number threshold as a first-line screening test. Patients with repeat numbers over the normal cut-off would then have a reflex test to determine precise repeat numbers in the premutation or full mutation range.

Recent newer methods, using techniques such as high-throughput PCR-based assays and mass spectrometry, which correctly detect expanded alleles in premutation and full mutation patients with a high degree of sensitivity,[33,34] show significant promise for reduction in cost with largely automated and rapid processes.[35]

COUNSELING ISSUES AND CHALLENGES

Whether or not universal screening is adopted, fragile X carrier testing and fetal diagnosis raises particular counseling challenges. Both the general public and primary care providers may be less familiar with FXS and its complex inheritance patterns. In patients identified as carriers, the genetic counseling is typically more difficult and may require more time than counseling for Down syndrome screening because patients are less familiar with the phenotype. All individuals identified as carriers of intermediate or premutation alleles should be referred for genetic counseling to properly convey risks for allele expansion (see **Table 2**) and to discuss possible future risks of fragile X–associated disease (see **Tables 3** and **4**). In the case of universal screening in the prenatal setting, this will necessarily lead to demands on resources, both in the primary care area and in specialty genetic services.

Previous studies of prenatal counseling in general suggest that women who participate in prenatal testing may experience higher levels of anxiety and may also be more likely to perceive their risk of having a child with a birth defect as greater than their actual risk.[36] In the case of FXS, the complexity of inheritance and possible outcomes, compounded by a general lack of background knowledge, impacts the individual's understanding and retention of critical information. Specifically, one study examining the uptake of fragile X carrier testing in a routine prenatal counseling setting noted that participants were generally unaware of FXS prior to screening. Retention of medical and genetic knowledge about FXS was limited, even though each participant was provided with counseling from an experienced prenatal genetic counselor and the participant population was highly educated.[27]

Patient understanding and retention of information illustrates a central concern in prenatal screening regarding the effectiveness of pretest counseling, particularly as the number of options for genetic screening increases. Although the medical provider or genetic counselor may strive to relay sufficient information for adequate informed consent, it is possible that many women will become overwhelmed with the number and complexity of disorders reviewed. This situation highlights the necessity for new educational tools and the reconsideration of modes of pre- and posttest counseling. Ideally, women should be given the opportunity to review information and consider the social and psychological issues related to fragile X carrier screening before screening or prenatal testing. It is essential that pretest information resources, including genetic counseling, be available to women considering screening. However, it seems clear that as the number of genetic diseases included in routine prenatal screening increases, the potential to deliver on pretest counseling becomes challenged.

Premutation Fragile X Allele Carriers and Adult-Onset Disease

Unlike other common population screening for autosomal recessive conditions, population screening for fragile X carriers will identify individuals at risk for adult-onset conditions. Specifically, detection of an expanded CGG repeat in the premutation range not only confers a risk to have offspring with FXS, but also confers a risk for FXPOI and FXTAS. Medical providers in the prenatal setting are not generally accustomed to this necessarily expanded focus in considering prenatal risk assessment. Pre- and posttest counseling must address the potential psychological and social impact of identifying an individual's risk for these adult-onset conditions.

Prenatal Identification of Male or Female Fetuses with a Premutation Fragile X Allele

If a woman is identified as a premutation carrier and she elects to undergo prenatal diagnostic testing for fragile X, she will have knowledge of the repeat size and gender of her fetus. As such, this individual may find that her fetus does not carry a full mutation but instead has inherited an allele in the premutation range. This scenario presents another counseling challenge in educating families about the implications and risks of a premutation allele. In particular, it involves the disclosure of information pertaining to the risk that the fetus may have to develop 2 adult-onset conditions, FXPOI and FXTAS.

Traditionally, when considering the implication of prenatal testing for adult-onset conditions such as these, careful analysis of the potential risks and benefits are made. Primarily, the direct medical benefit of identifying carriers prenatally should be explored. Other general benefits may include treatment and prevention, increased surveillance, reduction of uncertainty for the parent, and the option for knowledgeable family planning. Potential harms may include altered self image of the parent and child, distortion of parental perceptions of their child, increased parental anxiety or guilt, and altered expectations of the parent. Disclosure of carrier status to other at-risk family members is another consideration that deserves attention.[37]

It is clear that prenatal identification of a fetus with a premutation will allow parents to share important health information with these children at an appropriate age. As adults, these children can make informed decisions regarding pregnancy timing and desire for prenatal testing during their pregnancies. In addition, increased surveillance in adulthood may allow for earlier identification of individuals affected by FXTAS. However, it remains unclear whether any direct treatment or prevention options will be available.

At the same time, prenatal identification of offspring at risk for FXPOI and FXTAS may certainly alter the self image of the parent and child and lead to distortion of parental perceptions. This distortion may combine with increased parental anxiety and guilt to cause great distress for some women in the prenatal period. While it is beyond the scope of this article to fully analyze the impact of prenatal knowledge of fragile X allele status, these points are raised to emphasize the overall complexity of the disorder and the need to establish modes of patient and practitioner education to coincide with widespread screening.

Prenatal Identification of Female Fetuses with a Full Mutation

Prenatal prediction of the phenotype in female fetuses with a full mutation is limited; therefore, the identification of female fetuses with full mutations (>200) can pose a significant counseling challenge and a difficult set of choices for the parents. As anticipated for X-linked conditions, skewed X inactivation may modify the clinical phenotype of FXS in female carriers. If the percentage of active X chromosomes with the normal repeat allele is greater than the percentage of active X chromosomes with the full mutation allele, symptoms may be modified and less severe. Unfortunately, it is difficult to predict this activation ratio prenatally. In general, up to 50% of females with a full mutation allele will be significantly affected with cognitive and behavioral features of FXS.[7] Ultimately, for those women identified as carrying a female fetus with a full mutation, uncertainty about the resulting phenotype may certainly produce anxiety. This potential dilemma in counseling has led some to suggest that fetal diagnosis of fragile X be reserved only for male fetuses.[38]

Identification of Intermediate Fragile X Allele Carriers

Genetic counseling for individuals shown to have an intermediate allele has proven especially challenging. This repeat range (45–54), often referred to as the "gray zone," can cause moderate anxiety in patients because this result is not called "normal," and intermediate repeat sizes may be unstable and can expand in subsequent generations. To date there have been no reports of a CGG repeat of less than 56 expanding into a full mutation in a single generation (see earlier). However, despite possible patient anxiety in the setting of intermediate-zone repeats, offering invasive prenatal diagnosis to patients with intermediate-range repeats is not generally recommended, given the low probability that a CGG repeat of less than 55 will expand into a full mutation.[1] It should be noted that in light of reports of an intermediate allele expanding into a full mutation in 2 generations,[39] fragile X testing should be recommended to other family members within the same generation and to those in future generations to determine allele stability and identify individuals at risk for offspring with full mutations.

Although the risk of an expansion into a full mutation from an intermediate number of repeats is low, many women will still experience increased anxiety when identified as an intermediate allele carrier. To date, there are limited data on the psychological effects of identification of such an allele carrier. Ideally, this topic will continue to be explored, and appropriate protocols and educational resources will be developed to address the specific needs of these individuals. Until such resources are widespread, genetic counseling is recommended for all women identified as intermediate allele carriers.

FUTURE CONSIDERATIONS

Recent advances in mutation detection analysis either by high-throughput PCR, microarray, or sequencing-based technologies now offer the possibility to substantially increase the number of single gene diseases that can be tested in a single DNA sample and to potentially decrease the cost per condition screened. As noted earlier, the more disease screens offered in the prenatal setting will indeed challenge our ability to provide "traditional" pretest counseling. It is likely that other than providing appropriate pretest information (eg, print, Internet, video, group class), the classic model of face-to-face counseling might not be possible given the potential number of genetic counselors that will be available. More in line with pretest newborn screening methods, traditional genetic counseling may need to be reserved for those prenatal patients who are found to be a carrier. Even if screening panels do not target an increased number of conditions, reduction in cost for carrier screening for a disease such as fragile X and the adoption of widespread screening will likely prompt a change in the approach to counseling.

SUMMARY

Mutations of the FMR1 gene can affect the health of men, women, and their offspring, depending on the number of CGG repeats carried. Due to the variety of mutations and premutations found in carriers, and the resulting health implications, widespread prenatal screening for fragile X raises several counseling challenges. These challenges should be explored in greater detail to ensure the introduction of safe and effective widespread screening programs.

REFERENCES

1. Cronister A, Teicher J, Rohlfs EM, et al. Prevalence and instability of fragile X alleles: implications for offering fragile X prenatal diagnosis. Obstet Gynecol 2008;111(3):596–601.
2. Pesso R, Berkenstadt M, Cuckle H, et al. Screening for fragile X syndrome in women of reproductive age. Prenat Diagn 2000;20:611–4.
3. Hunter JE, Epstein MP, Tinker SW, et al. Fragile X-associated primary ovarian insufficiency: evidence for additional genetic contributions to severity. Genet Epidemiol 2008;32(6):553–9.

4. Leehey MA. Fragile X-associated tremor/ataxia syndrome: clinical phenotype, diagnosis, and treatment. J Investig Med 2009;57(8):830–6.

5. McConkie-Rosell A, Abrams L, Finucane B, et al. Recommendations from multi disciplinary focus groups on cascade testing and genetic counseling for fragile X associated disorders. J Genet Couns 2007;16:593–606.

6. Ennis S, Ward D, Murray A. Nonlinear association between CGG repeat number and age of menopause in FMR1 premutation carriers. Eur J Hum Genet 2006; 14(2):253–5.

7. Sherman S, Pletcher BA, Driscoll DA. Fragile X syndrome: diagnostic and carrier testing. Genet Med 2005;7:584–7.

8. Gleicher N, Weghofer A, Barad DH. A pilot study of premature ovarian senescence: I. Correlation of triple CGG repeats on the FMR1 gene to ovarian reserve parameters FSH and anti-Müllerian hormone. Fertil Steril 2009;91(5):1700–6.

9. Bretherick KL, Fluker MR, Robinson WP. FMR1 repeat sizes in the gray zone and high end of the normal range are associated with premature ovarian failure. Hum Genet 2005;117:376–82.

10. Bodega B, Bione S, Dalpra L, et al. Influence of intermediate and uninterrupted FMR1 CGG expansions in premature ovarian failure manifestation. Hum Reprod 2006;21:952–7.

11. Bennett CE, Conway GS, Macpherson JN, et al. Intermediate sized CGG repeats are not a common cause of idiopathic premature ovarian failure. Hum Reprod 2010;25(5):1335–8.

12. Hagerman RJ, Leehey M, Heinrichs W, et al. Intention tremor, parkinsonism and generalized brain atrophy in male carriers of fragile X. Neurology 2001;57:127–30.

13. Hagerman PJ, Hagerman RJ. The fragile-X premutation: a maturing perspective. Am J Hum Genet 2004;74:805–16.

14. Jacquemont S, Hagerman RJ, Leehey MA, et al. Penetrance of the fragile X-associated tremor/ataxia syndrome in a premutation carrier population. JAMA 2004; 291:460–9.

15. Coffey SM, Cook K, Tartaglia N, et al. Expanded clinical phenotype of women with the FMR1 premutation. Am J Med Genet A 2008;146A:1009–16.

16. Kronquist KE, Sherman SL, Spector EB. Clinical significance of tri-nucleotide repeats in fragile X testing: a clarification of American College of Medical Genetics guidelines. Genet Med 2008;10(11):845–7.

17. Nolin SL, Brown WT, Glicksman A, et al. Expansion of the fragile X CGG repeat in females with premutation or intermediate alleles. Am J Hum Genet 2003;72(2): 454–64.

18. Parniewski P, Staczek P. Review: molecular mechanisms of TRS instability. Adv Exp Med Biol 2002;516:1–25.

19. Jakupciak JP, Wells RD. Genetic instabilities of triplet repeat sequences by recombination. IUBMB Life 2000;50(6):355–9.

20. Fernandez-Carvajal I, Lopez Posadas B, Pan R, et al. Expansion of an FMR1 grey-zone allele to a full mutation in two generations. J Mol Diagn 2009;11(4): 306–10.

21. Tassone F, Beilina A, Carosi C, et al. Elevated FMR1 mRNA in premutation carriers is due to increased transcription. RNA 2007;13(4):555–62.

22. Sullivan AK, Marcus M, Epstein MP, et al. Association of FMR1 repeat size with ovarian dysfunction. Hum Reprod 2005;20:402–12.

23. Brouwer JR, Willemsen R, Oostra BA. The FMR1 gene and fragile X-associated tremor/ataxia syndrome. Am J Med Genet B Neuropsychiatr Genet 2009; 150B(6):782–98.

24. Spector EB, Kronquist KE. Fragile X: technical standards and guidelines. ACMG standards and guidelines for clinical genetics laboratories. 2005. Available at: http://www.ACMG.net. Accessed February 5, 2010.

25. McConkie-Rosell A, Finucan B, Cronister A, et al. Genetic counseling for fragile X syndrome: updated recommendations of the national society of genetic counselors. J Genet Couns 2005;14(4):246–70.

26. Cronister A, DiMaio M, Mahoney MJ, et al. Fragile X syndrome carrier screening in the prenatal genetic counseling setting. Genet Med 2005;7(4):246–50.

27. Fanos JH, Spangner KA, Musci TJ. Attitudes toward prenatal screening and testing for fragile X. Genet Med 2006;8(2):129–33.

28. Song FJ, Barton P, Sleightholme V, et al. Screening for fragile X syndrome: a literature review and modeling study. Health Technol Assess 2003;7:1–106.

29. Wilson JMG, Jungner G. Principles and practice of screening for disease. Geneva (Switzerland): World Health Organization; 1968. p. 165.

30. Khoury MJ, McCabe LL, McCabe ER. Population screening in the age of genomic medicine. N Engl J Med 2003;348:50–8.

31. Musci T. Screening for single gene genetic disease. Gynecol Obstet Invest 2005; 60:19–26.

32. Musci T, Caughey AB. Cost-effectiveness analysis of prenatal population-based fragile X carrier screening. Am J Obstet Gynecol 2005;192(6):1905–12 [discussion: 1912–5].

33. Lyon E, Yu P, Jama M, et al. A rapid PCR assay suitable for fragile X population screening [abstract 353]. In: Abstracts from the 16th Annual ACMG Annual Clinical Genetics Meeting Tampa (FL), March 25–29, 2009.

34. Strom CM, Huang D, Li Y, et al. Development of a novel, accurate, automated, rapid, high-throughput technique suitable for population-based carrier screening for fragile X syndrome. Genet Med 2007;9(4):199–207.

35. Dodds ED, Tassone F, Hagerman PJ, et al. Polymerase chain reaction, nuclease digestion, and mass spectrometry based assay for the trinucleotide repeat status of the fragile X mental retardation 1 gene. Anal Chem 2009;81(13):5533–40.

36. Tercyak KP, Bennett Johnson S, Roberts SF, et al. Psychological response to prenatal genetic counseling and amniocentesis. Patient Educ Couns 2001;43: 73–84.

37. The American Society of Human Genetics Board of Directors, The American College of Medical Genetics Board of Directors. Drafted by a subcommittee of the ASHG Social Issues Committees. In: Wilfond BS, Pelias MZ, Knoppers BM, et al. Genetic testing in children and adolescents, points to consider: ethical legal and psychosocial implications of (ACMG/ASHG). Am J Hum Genet 1995;57:1233–41.

38. Wald NJ, Morris JK. A new approach to antenatal screening for fragile X syndrome. Prenat Diagn 2003;23:345–51.

39. Terracciano A, Pomponi MG, Marino GM, et al. Expansion to full mutation of a FMR1 intermediate allele over two generations. Eur J Hum Genet 2004;12: 333–6.

Applications of Array Comparative Genomic Hybridization in Obstetrics

Gary Fruhman, MD[a], Ignatia B. Van den Veyver, MD[b],*

KEYWORDS

- Array comparative genomic hybridization • Prenatal diagnosis
- Fluorescence in situ hybridization • Cytogenetic diagnosis

A BRIEF HISTORY OF CYTOGENETICS

Modern cytogenetic techniques were first devised in the early 1950s, when it was accidentally discovered that a hypotonic solution can be used to spread chromosomes apart. Only then was the correct number of 46 chromosomes in a human confirmed.[1] Aneuploidy was recognized and the cytogenetic abnormality in Down syndrome, an extra chromosome 21, was first described in 1959.[2] During the late 1960s and early 1970s, Giemsa stains revealed the chromosomal G- and R-banding patterns, allowing pairing of homologous chromosomes during karyotype preparation. By examining G bands, skilled cytogeneticists can identify chromosomal deletions, duplications, inversions, and translocations, but the size of the abnormality needs to be a minimum of about 4 megabases (Mb; 4 million base pairs). Because culture of amniocytes or chorionic villi is required to obtain metaphases, 7 to 14 days are needed to obtain a karyotype in prenatal diagnosis.

Fluorescence in situ hybridization (FISH) was developed in the 1980s and has many applications.[3] In FISH, probes complementary to specific segments of DNA are labeled with fluorescent dyes and hybridized to DNA in nuclei of cells or metaphase spreads fixed to microscope slides (**Fig. 1**A). In prenatal diagnosis FISH is mostly used for rapid detection of trisomies 13, 18, or 21, and fetal gender determination by counting the number of signals of chromosome-specific probes. Cell culture is not necessary, and results can be obtained in as little as 24 hours. Syndromes caused by deletion or duplication of a specific segment of a chromosome, for example,

[a] Department of Molecular and Human Genetics, Baylor College of Medicine, 6621 Fannin Street CC 1560, Houston, TX 77030, USA
[b] Departments of Obstetrics and Gynecology and Molecular and Human Genetics, Baylor College of Medicine, 1709 Dryden, Suite 1100, Mail Stop BCM 610, Houston, TX 77030, USA
* Corresponding author.
E-mail address: iveyver@bcm.edu

Obstet Gynecol Clin N Am 37 (2010) 71–85
doi:10.1016/j.ogc.2010.02.001
0889-8545/10/$ – see front matter © 2010 Elsevier Inc. All rights reserved.

obgyn.theclinics.com

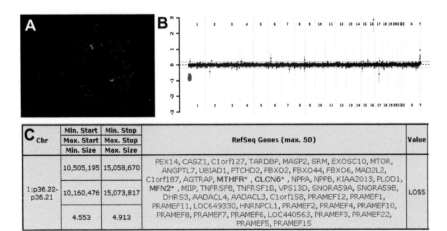

C Chr	Min. Start Max. Start Min. Size	Min. Stop Max. Stop Max. Size	RefSeq Genes (max. 50)	Value
1:p36.22- p36.21	10,505,195	15,058,670	PEX14, CASZ1, C1orf127, TARDBP, MASP2, SRM, EXOSC10, MTOR, ANGPTL7, UBIAD1, PTCHD2, FBXO2, FBXO44, FBXO6, MAD2L2, C1orf187, AGTRAP, **MTHFR*** , **CLCN6*** , NPPA, NPPB, KIAA2013, PLOD1, MFN2* , MIIP, TNFRSF8, TNFRSF1B, VPS13D, SNORA59A, SNORA59B, DHRS3, AADACL4, AADACL3, C1orf158, PRAMEF12, PRAMEF1, PRAMEF11, LOC649330, HNRNPCL1, PRAMEF2, PRAMEF4, PRAMEF10, PRAMEF8, PRAMEF7, PRAMEF6, LOC440563, PRAMEF3, PRAMEF22, PRAMEF5, PRAMEF15	LOSS
	10,160,476	15,073,817		
	4.553	4.913		

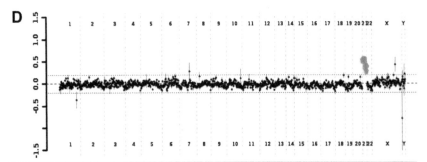

E Chr	Min. Start Max. Start Min. Size	Min. Stop Max. Stop Max. Size	RefSeq Genes (max. 50)	Value
21:q11.2-q22.3	14,445,069	46,913,787	LIPI, RBM11, HSPA13, SAMSN1, NRIP1, USP25, C21orf34, CXADR, BTG3, C21orf91, CHODL, PRSS7, NCAM2, MRPL39, JAM2, ATP5J, GABPA, APP, CYYR1, ADAMTS1, ADAMTS5, N6AMT1, ZNF294, RWDD2B, USP16, CCT8, C21orf7, BACH1, GRIK1, CLDN17, CLDN8, KRTAP24-1, KRTAP25-1, KRTAP26-1, KRTAP27-1, KRTAP23-1, KRTAP13-2, KRTAP13-1, KRTAP13-3, KRTAP13-4, KRTAP15-1, KRTAP19-1, KRTAP19-2, KRTAP19-3, KRTAP19-4, KRTAP19-5, KRTAP19-6, KRTAP19-7, KRTAP6-3, KRTAP6-2	GAIN
	1	46,944,323		
	32.469	46.944		

Fig. 1. Examples of FISH and aCGH results. (*A*) FISH of a patient with a deletion on 1p36. Note the missing red signals from the 1p36 region on one of the chromosomes 1, which are identified by the control green signals. (*B*) Results of aCGH analysis for the same deletion. The x-axis shows the order of probes from chromosomes 1 to 22, X, and Y. The y-axis shows the signal intensities of the hybridization signals to reference oligonucleotides of patient DNA compared with reference DNA on a logarithmic scale. The deletion is identified by deviation of the hybridization signals (*red dots*) from the baseline (*black dots*). (*C*) Information regarding the chromosomal abnormality, including minimum and maximum sizes of these abnormalities. (*D*) aCGH result of a patient with trisomy 21. The green dots indicate the gain of all clones on chromosome 21 over baseline. (*E*) Information regarding the gene content of the extra chromosome 21.

Velocardiofacial/DiGeorge syndrome caused by deletion of the 22q11.2 region, can be detected using locus-specific probes.[4] FISH can be performed on nondividing interphase cells or on metaphase spreads. Using the latter, the chromosomal location of extra copies of a specific region in duplications or unbalanced translocations can be demonstrated. Specialized subtelomeric probes can be used to identify small terminal (telomere) deletions of chromosomes, while mixtures of probes covering entire chromosomes allow for chromosome "painting," which aids in detailed identification of translocations but is a cumbersome technique seldom used in prenatal diagnosis.

PRINCIPLES OF ARRAY-BASED COMPARATIVE GENOMIC HYBRIDIZATION

One of the major limitations of FISH in the diagnosis of chromosomal deletion and duplication syndromes is that the clinician must suspect a specific diagnosis, caused by changes of a particular chromosome or chromosomal region, to request the appropriate FISH test. This situation is not practical for broad diagnoses such as developmental delay, mental retardation, or autism with or without dysmorphism or minor anomalies. Over the past 10 years, a diagnostic revolution has taken place with the advent of array-based comparative genomic hybridization (aCGH).[5] This technology has the capacity to interrogate the entire genome for copy number changes caused by deletions, duplications, aneuploidy, or unbalanced translocations in a single assay, down to as small a size as that of a single exon on some platforms.

In the standard (non–array-based) method of comparative genomic hybridization, the binding of differentially labeled DNA from 2 different sources to metaphase spreads of reference genomic DNA from an individual with a normal karyotype is compared, with a resolution only minimally better than that of a standard karyotype.[6] This method has now been replaced by aCGH whereby the 2 sources of DNA are cohybridized to thousands of reference DNA fragments that are ordered on a solid surface such as a microscope slide.

Initial aCGH platforms were composed of multiple bacterial artificial clones (BACs) that contain inserts of reference DNA of 100 to 200 kilobases (kb) long. The number of BAC clones and covered regions on such arrays increased with subsequent versions, resulting in development of clinical "targeted arrays" covering over 100 genomic disorders with less dense "backbone coverage" for the rest of the genome.[7] Although still in use by some, BAC arrays are now being replaced by arrays of much shorter oligonucleotides, each between 25 and 80 nucleotides in length, depending on the specific platforms (see **Fig. 1B–E**). When designed for clinical diagnostic applications, these arrays remain targeted with concentrated coverage in known disease-causing regions of the genome and more limited coverage of areas of the genome for which copy number variants are not (yet) known to cause human disease or are of uncertain significance. The most recently developed version of such a "targeted array" for clinical diagnosis at the authors' institution contains 180,000 different oligonucleotides providing exon-by-exon coverage of more than 1700 disease-causing genes, 700 microRNAs, and the mitochondrial genome; it also includes "backbone" coverage of the entire genome at an average interoligonucleotide spacing of 30 kb. Most clinical diagnostic laboratories use various iterations of similar targeted platforms, but others have advocated the use of high-resolution "nontargeted" genome-wide arrays.[8] These arrays are also increasingly used as supplementary diagnostic tools for the most challenging cases.

In the "comparative" aCGH approach, sample (patient) DNA and a reference DNA are fluorescently labeled in different colors, and equal amounts are cohybridized to the array for several hours.[7] The chosen reference DNA is typically of the same gender of the sample DNA, but some have advocated the use of gender-mismatched DNA, or even DNA from an individual with a 47,XXY karyotype (Klinefelter syndrome) to improve the detection of sex chromosome abnormalities.[9] After a series of washing steps the array is scanned, and the intensity of each label is detected and interpreted using specialized software (**Fig. 2**). If the fluorescence intensity of the patient sample at certain oligonucleotides on the array is greater than that of the reference sample, there is a gain of copy number (eg, duplication or trisomy) for the region represented by those oligonucleotides (see **Figs. 1B–E** and **2**). By contrast, if the fluorescence intensity of the patient sample is less than that of the reference, there is a loss of copy number (eg, deletion or monosomy) for that region (see **Figs. 1B–E** and **2**). When the signal intensities are equal, there is no change in copy number. It should be noted that these signal intensities are interpreted using complex bioinformatics tools that take into account the values at each probe within the context of the entire array. Each commercial array and individual laboratory often apply customized software for these calculations, and subtle abnormalities such as mosaicism may have variable detection rates depending on the platforms used.

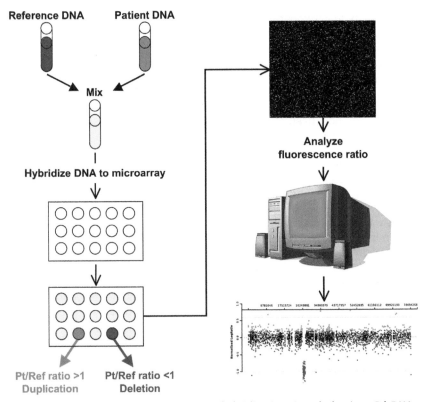

Fig. 2. Principle of array comparative genomic hybridization. Sample (patient; Pt) DNA and reference (Ref) DNA are each labeled with different fluorescent dyes. Equal amounts of sample and reference DNA are mixed, and allowed to hybridize with the oligonucleotide probes on the slide. If there is less patient DNA compared with reference DNA at a given location, a weaker signal from the sample DNA is emitted and this is interpreted as a copy number loss. If there is more patient DNA compared with the reference DNA at a given location it emits a stronger signal, which is interpreted as a copy number gain.

THE BASIS OF SINGLE NUCLEOTIDE POLYMORPHISM ARRAYS

Alternative platforms to the traditional "comparative" aCGH are based on single-sample hybridization to arrays that were initially designed for single nucleotide polymorphism (SNP) detection. SNPs are single-nucleotide changes in a given sequence of DNA (eg, ATAACGTA to ACAACGTA) that occur in at least 1% of the population and are present approximately every 100 to 300 base pairs. Most SNPs have no known direct clinical effect, but alternate alleles at certain SNPs may impact predisposition to or severity of common diseases, as well as drug metabolism. Soon after the development of arrays designed for genome-wide screens of the alleles of thousands of SNPs in a single assay, it was discovered that modification of data analysis tools and probe optimization of such arrays also made them useful for identification of copy number variation.[10]

Currently used versions of SNP arrays can contain more than a million reference oligonucleotides. In one approach, sample DNA is annealed to short oligonucleotides on the array followed by a single base extension with single nucleotides (A, C, G, or T) complementary to the DNA sequence carrying a different fluorescent tag. Specialized software detects the fluorescence intensity and identity of each base at a given location, such that copy number losses and gains (deletions and duplications) can be detected from this combined information. Because the SNP array provides information about alleles of single bases, "absence of heterozygosity" (AOH) without copy number loss or gain (ie, copy-neutral AOH) can also be detected. This situation occurs due to the presence of 2 identical alleles at a given position, which can occur if there is uniparental isodisomy whereby both alleles were inherited from the same parent, or if 2 identical alleles are inherited from a common ancestor, as in consanguinity whereby typically multiple large regions of copy-neutral AOH are present (**Fig. 3**).

Despite these additional benefits compared with the "comparative" aCGH, SNP arrays can be less sensitive with more background noise, causing difficulty with interpreting results. The authors therefore still use the aCGH approach as the first-line tool for copy number analysis in clinical diagnosis, but as technology improves, SNP-based arrays may replace comparative aCGH platforms.

USE OF ACGH FOR DISCOVERY AND DELINEATION OF GENOMIC DISORDERS

As demonstrated by the examples in this article, aCGH has been instrumental for the improved characterization of known genetic disorders and the discovery of novel ones. One of the first was the discovery of the molecular basis of CHARGE syndrome (Coloboma, Heart disease, Atresia of the choanae, Retarded growth and development, Genital hypoplasia, and Ear anomalies). Two patients with this disorder had 8q12 deletions detected by aCGH; this prompted the sequencing of genes in this region, ultimately pointing to mutations in the CHD7 gene as the cause of most CHARGE syndrome cases.[11] aCGH was also instrumental in the authors' laboratory for the discovery that mutations in PORCN cause focal dermal hypoplasia.[12,13] Monosomy 1p36, associated with developmental delay, mental retardation, dysmorphic features, hypotonia, and hearing defects, is usually caused by a terminal deletion of this region. However, aCGH has uncovered previously unascertained interstitial deletions and complex rearrangements resulting in monosomy 1p36.[14] In addition to expanding the knowledge base of known rare genetic syndromes, research over the past 10 years has implicated an ever-growing number of genomic microduplications and microdeletions in the etiology of more common disorders, mental retardation, and unspecified dysmorphism. Some examples include the discovery that a microduplication of 17p11.2, affecting the same region that is deleted in Smith-Magenis

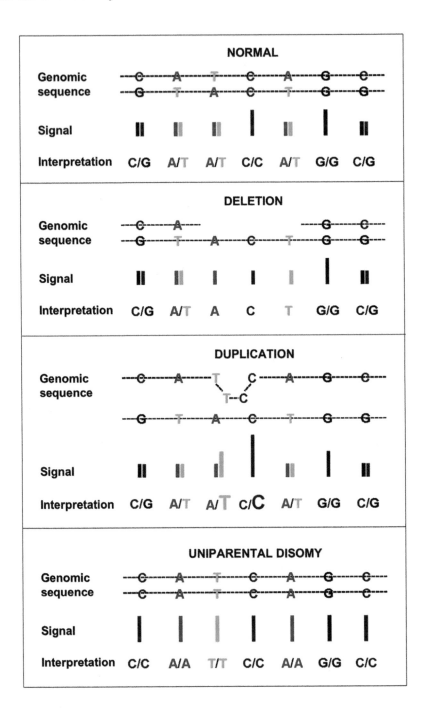

syndrome, causes Potocki-Lupski syndrome.[15,16] Other examples include the association of microdeletions at 17q21.3 with learning disabilities and developmental delay,[17] the association of 1q21.1 microdeletions with microcephaly, developmental delay, and mental retardation,[18,19] and the association of microdeletions at 16p11.2 with autism.[20] A duplication in the Xq28 region containing the Rett syndrome gene, *MECP2*, was discovered and characterized using aCGH as a relatively common cause of autism and mental retardation in males.[21] Most recently, microdeletions of *CHRNA7* located on 15q13.3, have been implicated in the majority of neurodevelopmental phenotypes associated with 15q13.3 syndrome.[22] It is of note that most of these conditions, as well as most other known deletion and duplication syndromes, would not present with any specific prenatal risk factors or characteristic ultrasound findings.

CLINICAL DIAGNOSTIC USE AND GENERAL BENEFITS OF ACGH

Karyotype and aCGH will both detect aneuploidy, unbalanced translocations, deletions, and duplications if the size is at least 4 Mb (**Fig. 4**). However, aCGH has much higher resolution and therefore sensitivity, and can detect very small copy number gains or losses, typically as small as 50 to 100 kb, but detection even of a single exon is possible (see **Fig. 4**). It has been reported that with aCGH, clinically significant copy number abnormalities can be detected in 5% to 8% of pediatric and adult patients with developmental disability, dysmorphic features, or congenital anomalies, who had a previously reported "normal" karyotype.[23] With improvements in technology and use of more sensitive arrays, this number continues to increase and is currently estimated to be around 10%, ranging from 8% to 17%.[24] Furthermore, because cell cultures are not needed for aCGH, the turnaround time from sample submission to diagnosis is usually shorter compared with traditional cytogenetic methods.

GENERAL LIMITATIONS OF ACGH

Although aCGH is more sensitive than a karyotype for the detection of small deletions and copy number gains, the exact size of the detected deletion or duplication cannot always be determined, as it depends on the spacing between the first flanking probes and the deleted probes for a particular region. Hence, diagnostic laboratories issuing aCGH results will often report a minimum and maximum size of the cytogenetic abnormality.

Other limitations of aCGH include the inability to diagnose totally balanced structural chromosomal abnormalities such as balanced translocations or inversions. Of note, with aCGH use it has become clear that often such "apparently balanced" rearrangements seen on karyotype are in fact unbalanced and accompanied by loss, or sometimes gain, of genomic material at the translocation breakpoints that was not

---

Fig. 3. Principle of copy number analysis using SNP arrays. The top row in each panel represents a theoretical example of an individual's SNP alleles at contiguous locations, with expected signal intensities from the SNP array analysis below it, followed by the interpretation of the obtained signals. Theoretical expected results for different scenarios: normal copy number, deletion (copy number loss), duplication (copy number gain), and uniparental disomy are shown in respective panels. Note that in the uniparental disomy example, all alleles show a strong signal emitted from 2 bases that are the same. This phenomenon is called "absence of heterozygosity," in contrast to "loss of heterozygosity" in case of a deletion; this can also be seen if there is consanguinity with extensive regions of homozygosity by descent.

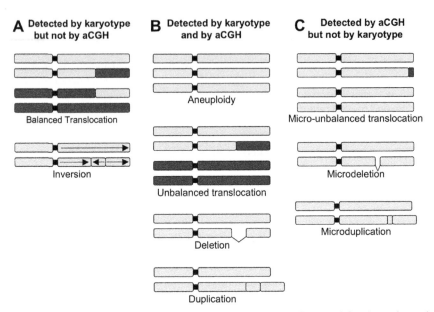

A Detected by karyotype but not by aCGH

Balanced Translocation

Inversion

B Detected by karyotype and by aCGH

Aneuploidy

Unbalanced translocation

Deletion

Duplication

C Detected by aCGH but not by karyotype

Micro-unbalanced translocation

Microdeletion

Microduplication

Fig. 4. Comparison of abnormalities detected by karyotype and aCGH. (*A*) Balanced translocations and inversions can be detected by karyotype analysis, but not by aCGH. (B) Aneuploidy, unbalanced translocations, and deletions or duplications greater than 4 Mb can be detected by both karyotype and aCGH. (C) Microdeletions, microduplications, or microunbalanced translocations, smaller than 4 Mb, can be detected by aCGH but not by karyotype.

apparent on karyotype.[25] Because aCGH cannot specify the exact location of a detected copy number gain, in certain cases a karyotype or FISH will be necessary to further characterize it.[7] For example, if there is a gain of an entire chromosome 21, only the karyotype will discern between trisomy 21 and an unbalanced Robertsonian translocation, which has relevance for recurrence risk counseling. Reported smaller copy number gains are commonly duplications within the affected region, but without a karyotype or FISH it is impossible to distinguish these from material of the duplicated region having inserted at other chromosomal locations. aCGH cannot easily detect polyploidy, unless the karyotype is 69, XXY, where the sex chromosome imbalance will trigger further investigation for this possible diagnosis. aCGH by design will not detect point mutations, responsible for many Mendelian disorders such as cystic fibrosis. However, this is being developed using SNP-based platforms and may become clinical reality in future years. Finally, although aCGH can detect mosaicism for structural genomic abnormalities or marker chromosomes, very low levels may remain undetected. Because of its special relevance to prenatal diagnosis, this is discussed in the following section.

THE PRENATAL EXPERIENCE: SUCCESSES AND LIMITATIONS

One of the first studies of aCGH analysis on prenatal samples was reported by Rickman and colleagues[26] in 2005. These investigators blindly studied 30 uncultured samples of fetal cells obtained from 1 to 2 mL of amniotic fluid and from chorionic villus samples that had known chromosomal abnormalities confirmed by karyotype. Each sample was interrogated on a small custom array optimized for prenatal diagnosis that contained 600 probes, and in parallel on an array with clones spaced

1 Mb apart spanning the entire genome. Known anomalies were correctly detected with the custom array in 29 of 30 samples, but only in 22 of 30 with the genome-wide array. Larrabee and colleagues[27] found that amniotic fluid supernatant contains a significant amount of cell-free fetal DNA. However, when amniotic fluid supernatant was analyzed on an array with 287 clones, anomalies were detected in only 4 of 9 known samples. In 2006, Sahoo and colleagues[28] reported a series of 98 women undergoing invasive prenatal diagnosis who agreed to have an aCGH test in addition to the standard G-banded karyotype. The karyotype detected 4 cases of trisomy 21 and 1 unbalanced translocation of chromosomes 3 and 7. aCGH detected these abnormalities, as well as copy number variants in 42 other cases. Thirty of the copy number variants were known to be benign variants while 12 required further parental testing for optimal interpretation; most of these were also interpreted as benign. In 2008, Shaffer and colleagues[29] compared the detection rate of prenatal and postnatal targeted aCGH. In this study, the indications for the prenatal array included advanced maternal age, abnormal ultrasound, family history of genetic disease or chromosomal abnormality, further workup for chromosomal abnormalities detected on karyotype, and parental anxiety. Postnatal aCGH was obtained from patients younger than 3 months who presented with an abnormal family history, dysmorphic features, developmental delay, or other abnormal features. Compared with 156 of 1375 (11.4%) postnatal cases, only 2 of 151 (1.3%) prenatal cases showed a clinically significant change. Subsequently, Van den Veyver and colleagues[30] reviewed 300 cases of clinical prenatal diagnosis using aCGH from samples obtained from women already undergoing invasive prenatal diagnosis for karyotype analysis for standard indications. Indications included abnormal maternal serum screening, advanced maternal age, fetal abnormalities detected by ultrasound, parental anxiety, further characterization of marker chromosomes, or another karyotype abnormality. Of these, 242 cases had normal results and 58 showed copy number variants. Forty of these were interpreted to be of no clinical significance. Of the other 18, including whole chromosome aneuploidy, marker chromosomes, and results of unknown clinical significance, 10 copy number variants were not detected on fetal karyotype analysis. aCGH yielded clinically relevant additional information in 7 of 300 cases (2.3%), including the marker chromosomes mentioned above, the discovery of a 9q34 deletion in an apparently balanced translocation, an 800+ kb deletion in 15q26.3, and a case of TAR (Thrombocytopenia with Absent Radius) syndrome discovered after aCGH showed a deletion in 1q21.1. Six months later, Coppinger and colleagues[31] reviewed 182 prenatal aCGH results. In this study the aCGH was done for a family history of a chromosomal abnormality, abnormal ultrasound, abnormal maternal serum screening, parental anxiety, and advanced maternal age. Significant chromosomal alterations were noted in 7 cases, of which 2 were also identified by karyotype analysis. The diagnostic yield of aCGH was 5 out of 182 (2.7%), similar to the 2.3% found in the Van den Veyver study.[30] One detected abnormality was an unbalanced translocation, and 4 were significant copy number variants. Copy number variants thought to be benign were noted in 16 cases (8.8%).

Small supernumerary marker chromosomes (sSMC) are structurally abnormal small chromosomes that cannot be identified or characterized unambiguously by standard cytogenetic techniques.[32] While FISH can help identify the origin of sSMC, prior knowledge of the region likely to be involved is required. In contrast, aCGH can detect and characterize the origin of sSMCs as a copy number gain for the pericentromeric genomic region present in the sSMC, if it is represented on the array used.[33] One group reported the development and validation on 20 samples of a high-density pericentromeric BAC microarray for this purpose.[34] Previously known sSMCs were detected in 15 cases, and their origin and size determined for some of them. Smaller sSMCs that remain undetected are more likely to contain only repetitive DNA, and are therefore of lesser clinical importance. In other cases, the level of mosaicism may be below the sensitivity of the array technology. Karyotype may not detect such mosaic sSMCs well either, because cells with markers may be less likely successfully stimulated to divide in order to obtain a karyotype.[35] aCGH has also been used to identify sSMCs in prenatal samples,[30] and Gruchy and colleagues[36] reviewed 20 prenatal cases with sSMCs diagnosed without the aid of aCGH, concluding that aCGH would not have added new data in 9, but would have improved diagnostic accuracy in 6 and identified the origin of the sSMC in 5.

Mosaicism is the presence of more than one genetically distinct cell line in an organism.[37] Mosaicism can be detected using aCGH, and studies have shown a frequency of approximately 0.4% in the pediatric population.[35] Mosaicism is of particular concern in prenatal diagnosis, especially with chorionic villus sampling (CVS), where confined placental mosaicism can be found 1% to 2% of the time; mosaicism in amniocentesis occurs between 0.1% and 0.3% of the time.[38,39] aCGH was initially thought not to be sensitive enough to detect chromosomal mosaicism if less than 15% to 30% of the cells have the abnormal karyotype.[7] However, more recent studies have shown that the detection rate in some cases is higher than that of a conventional karyotype on DNA from blood samples[35] because for prenatal aCGH, chorionic villi or amniocytes can be directly analyzed, without prior culture in most cases.[40] Because the mosaic abnormal cell line may have a growth disadvantage in culture, true fetal or placental mosaicism may actually be detected at a higher rate with aCGH than with conventional karyotyping.[41]

THE ROLE OF ACGH IN THE CYTOGENETIC ANALYSIS OF PREGNANCY LOSS

It has been well established that 15% of all clinically established pregnancies result in a spontaneous abortion and about 50% to 60% of failed first-trimester pregnancies have chromosomal abnormalities, including aneuploidy or polyploidy, de novo unbalanced translocations, or unbalanced translocations inherited from a parent with a balanced translocation.[42] Especially in cases of recurrent miscarriage, conventional cytogenetic testing is often done on the products of conception to determine if a cytogenetic abnormality caused the pregnancy loss, but culture failure and maternal cell contamination overgrowing fetal cells in culture are common. aCGH does not require actively dividing cells and overcomes these limitations. In the first reported study, 41 products of conception samples were karyotyped and concurrently analyzed by aCGH.[41] Results (24 normal and 13 abnormal) were concordant in 37 cases, but aCGH detected abnormalities in 4 cases that were not seen on the karyotype. Benkhalifa and colleagues[42] evaluated products of conception using aCGH from 26 first-trimester miscarriages that could not be evaluated using conventional cytogenetic methods. Fifteen had an abnormal profile, of which 4 showed a double aneuploidy and 5 had autosomal monosomy, both rarely reported findings with conventional cytogenetic studies. In another study, 2 submicroscopic deletions were found in 20 CVS samples from spontaneous abortions with normal karyotypes that had subsequent aCGH analysis; one finding was detectable but not initially found on the karyotype analysis because of maternal cell contamination.[43] Recently, another group reported on the benefits of flow cytometry and aCGH compared with karyotype.[44] In this study, karyotype could not be obtained in 28 of 100 cases while aCGH was not possible in only 2. Chromosome analysis revealed 17 abnormal karyotypes, but aCGH combined with flow cytometry found abnormalities in 26 samples. Finally, in a recent study patients with fetal demises underwent embryoscopy followed by CVS and karyotype analysis if a fetus had a structural abnormality. If there was a normal karyotype, aCGH testing followed, which revealed abnormalities in 5 of 17 such patients.[45]

GENETIC COUNSELING

The importance and complexity of genetic counseling for aCGH-based clinical diagnosis cannot be underestimated. Important issues to address were recently described in detail and are reviewed briefly here.[46] In the pediatric or adult population, aCGH analysis is usually recommended for birth defects, dysmorphic fetures, developmental delay or neurobehavioral abnormalities. Prenatally, aCGH is currently mostly performed if there is a family history of a genetic disease, if serum screening tests are abnormal, or if abnormal ultrasound findings are noted. However, it is increasingly offered to women undergoing invasive prenatal diagnosis for standard indications, such as an elevated risk for Down syndrome, and is also requested by women at no known risk factors for fetal chromosomal abnormalities. In fact, many of the structural chromosomal abnormalities that are detectable by aCGH are not known to be associated with advanced maternal age or abnormal results on maternal serum analytes.

Pretest counseling, especially when done prenatally, should include a generalized discussion of chromosomes and genes, a description of the test, and possible outcomes. Pretest counseling should briefly review the benefits and limitations of aCGH compared with routinely used diagnostic tests such as karyotype and FISH, and highlight the abnormalities it can and cannot detect. As with other prenatal diagnostic tests, patients should be aware that not all findings will be of well-defined clinical significance and that sometimes additional testing may be needed to clarify a detected copy number abnormality. The parents should be prepared to donate a blood sample at the time of fetal sample collection so that an abnormality detected in the fetal sample can rapidly be verified on parental DNA to determine if it is de novo or inherited from a healthy parent. A signed informed consent document for the testing and summarizing of the information, with a copy retained in the medical record, is desirable. More detailed information about aCGH can be made available to the families who desire to do further research.

Providers with genetics training should ideally communicate abnormal aCGH results to families, explain the finding in lay terms, discuss the current knowledge of its association with a known genetic disorder, and review the phenotype of the detected disorder. In some situations, further laboratory testing may be necessary to determine the extent and the clinical consequence of the abnormality, and the role of these tests should be explained to the family. As with every prenatal diagnostic test, it is important to highlight that negative results, while reassuring, do not unequivocally rule out a genetic or developmental disorder. Clinical aCGH testing does not interrogate every part of the genome, and current methods are also not designed to detect point mutations causing Mendelian disorders like cystic fibrosis or triplet repeat amplifications that cause diseases like Fragile X syndrome.

Copy number variants of unknown clinical significance are sometimes detected by aCGH, resulting in the need to communicate some degree of uncertainty in the counseling about the predicted phenotype, especially in the prenatal setting, where a phenotype may not be apparent in the fetus. Findings of uncertain clinical significance have been reported in prenatal aCGH series in approximately 0.5% to 1% of cases,[29-31] and can increase anxiety for patients and uncertainty about their reproductive options, for example, whether to continue or terminate a pregnancy. Pretest counseling about this small possibility for a result of uncertain significance will help prepare the parents. As more data are collected and clinical presentations are correlated with molecular findings over time, cataloging of clinically significant and apparently benign polymorphic variants will advance and the number of cases with uncertain results should diminish. Various efforts are currently underway to catalog copy number variants with clinical phenotypes that can be consulted as a reference when an aCGH result of unclear clinical significance is obtained. Two examples of such databases include the Database of Genomic Variants (DGV), located at http://projects.tcag.ca/variation/ and the DatabasE of Chromosomal Imbalance and Phenotype in Humans using Ensembl Resources (DECIPHER), located at https://decipher.sanger.ac.uk/application/. It is also important to consider that findings of uncertain or unknown clinical significance are regularly found with other commonly used prenatal diagnostic modalities such as ultrasound. For example, findings of isolated mild ventriculomegaly or agenesis of the corpus callosum are not uncommon, and while overall numbers of their association with suboptimal developmental outcome are available, often this cannot be accurately predicted in individual cases.

SUMMARY

The use of aCGH as a clinical diagnostic tool for detecting prenatal chromosomal abnormalities is becoming more widespread. aCGH can detect all unbalanced chromosomal abnormalities seen on a karyotype and chromosomal deletions or duplications that are much smaller than what can be detected using routine cytogenetic analysis, with a potentially faster turnaround time. aCGH performs well for detecting marker chromosomes and mosaicism if a sufficient percentage of the cells are affected, and has shown clear benefit for detecting chromosomal abnormalities in products of conception. aCGH will not reveal completely balanced structural abnormalities, performs suboptimally for polyploidy, and has not yet been optimized for clinical prenatal diagnosis of point mutations, but future potential for this can be anticipated.

Whether aCGH should be offered to all pregnant women or only in certain clinical scenarios, such as when fetal anomalies are detected by ultrasound, remains an issue of debate.[47] Surveys indicate that women want to obtain as much information about the fetus as possible, but have reservations about invasive prenatal diagnostic procedures.[48] In November 2009, the American College of Obstetrics and Gynecology released a committee opinion stating that conventional karyotyping should remain the principal mode of cytogenetic evaluation of prenatal samples, and that aCGH can be offered in specific cases, including abnormal anatomic findings on ultrasound with a normal karyotype or the evaluation of a fetal demise.[49] Smaller studies revealed that approximately 2% of fetuses with abnormal ultrasound findings will have clinically significant aCGH results.[30] A multicenter study sponsored by the National Institutes of Health evaluating aCGH for prenatal diagnosis that will address some of these issues is currently underway.

KEY POINTS

- Array-based comparative genomic hybridization is a powerful new technology for genome-wide detection of unbalanced chromosomal abnormalities, such as copy number variants, deletion and duplication syndromes, unbalanced translocations, and aneuploidy, but it cannot detect balanced chromosomal abnormalities.
- The resolution of aCGH is much higher than that of conventional karyotyping, which only detects chromosomal abnormalities of minimum 4 Mb.

- Copy number variants have been implicated in the etiology of birth defects, mental retardation, and other common disorders such as autism and schizophrenia.
- Until now there have only been a limited number of studies on the role of aCGH for prenatal diagnosis, but the results have been promising.
- While potential detection of copy number variants of uncertain or known clinical significance by aCGH is an important concern of health care providers, current studies suggest that these results occur only between 0.5% and 1% of the time.
- The potential for results of unknown clinical significance are a reality of other commonly used prenatal diagnostic modalities, such as ultrasound.
- Genetic counseling to discuss the benefits and limitations of aCGH and informed consent for testing are recommended before obtaining a sample for aCGH analysis.
- A large multicenter trial sponsored by the National Institutes of Health is currently underway to evaluate the benefit of aCGH for prenatal diagnosis.

REFERENCES

1. Gilgenkrantz S, Rivera EM. The history of cytogenetics. Portraits of some pioneers. Ann Genet 2003;46(4):433–42.
2. Lejeune J, Turpin R, Gautier M. [Chromosomic diagnosis of mongolism]. Arch Fr Pediatr 1959;16:962–3 [in French].
3. Trask BJ. Human cytogenetics: 46 chromosomes, 46 years and counting. Nat Rev Genet 2002;3(10):769–78.
4. Desmaze C, Prieur M, Amblard F, et al. Physical mapping by FISH of the DiGeorge critical region (DGCR): involvement of the region in familial cases. Am J Hum Genet 1993;53(6):1239–49.
5. Beaudet AL, Belmont JW. Array-based DNA diagnostics: let the revolution begin. Annu Rev Med 2008;59:113–29.
6. Kirchhoff M, Rose H, Lundsteen C. High resolution comparative genomic hybridisation in clinical cytogenetics. J Med Genet 2001;38(11):740–4.
7. Cheung SW, Shaw CA, Yu W, et al. Development and validation of a CGH microarray for clinical cytogenetic diagnosis. Genet Med 2005;7(6):422–32.
8. Veltman JA, de Vries BB. Diagnostic genome profiling: unbiased whole genome or targeted analysis? J Mol Diagn 2006;8(5):534–7 [discussion: 537–9].
9. Ballif BC, Kashork CD, Saleki R, et al. Detecting sex chromosome anomalies and common triploidies in products of conception by array-based comparative genomic hybridization. Prenat Diagn 2006;26(4):333–9.
10. Rauch A, Ruschendorf F, Huang J, et al. Molecular karyotyping using an SNP array for genomewide genotyping. J Med Genet 2004;41(12):916–22.
11. Vissers LE, van Ravenswaaij CM, Admiraal R, et al. Mutations in a new member of the chromodomain gene family cause CHARGE syndrome. Nat Genet 2004; 36(9):955–7.
12. Grzeschik KH, Bornholdt D, Oeffner F, et al. Deficiency of PORCN, a regulator of Wnt signaling, is associated with focal dermal hypoplasia. Nat Genet 2007;39(7): 833–5.
13. Wang X, Reid Sutton V, Omar Peraza-Llanes J, et al. Mutations in X-linked PORCN, a putative regulator of Wnt signaling, cause focal dermal hypoplasia. Nat Genet 2007;39(7):836–8.
14. Gajecka M, Mackay KL, Shaffer LG. Monosomy 1p36 deletion syndrome. Am J Med Genet C Semin Med Genet 2007;145(4):346–56.

15. Potocki L, Bi W, Treadwell-Deering D, et al. Characterization of Potocki-Lupski syndrome (dup(17) (p11.2p11.2)) and delineation of a dosage-sensitive critical interval that can convey an autism phenotype. Am J Hum Genet 2007;80(4):633–49.

16. Greenberg F, Guzzetta V, Montes de Oca-Luna R, et al. Molecular analysis of the Smith-Magenis syndrome: a possible contiguous-gene syndrome associated with del(17) (p11.2). Am J Hum Genet 1991;49(6):1207–18.

17. Sharp AJ, Hansen S, Selzer RR, et al. Discovery of previously unidentified genomic disorders from the duplication architecture of the human genome. Nat Genet 2006;38(9):1038–42.

18. Mefford HC, Sharp AJ, Baker C, et al. Recurrent rearrangements of chromosome 1q21.1 and variable pediatric phenotypes. N Engl J Med 2008;359(16): 1685–99.

19. Brunetti-Pierri N, Berg JS, Scaglia F, et al. Recurrent reciprocal 1q21.1 deletions and duplications associated with microcephaly or macrocephaly and developmental and behavioral abnormalities. Nat Genet 2008;40(12):1466–71.

20. Kumar RA, KaraMohamed S, Sudi J, et al. Recurrent 16p11.2 microdeletions in autism. Hum Mol Genet 2008;17(4):628–38.

21. del Gaudio D, Fang P, Scaglia F, et al. Increased MECP2 gene copy number as the result of genomic duplication in neurodevelopmentally delayed males. Genet Med 2006;8(12):784–92.

22. Shinawi M, Schaaf CP, Bhatt SS, et al. A small recurrent deletion within 15q13.3 is associated with a range of neurodevelopmental phenotypes. Nat Genet 2009; 41(12):1269–71.

23. Lu X, Shaw CA, Patel A, et al. Clinical implementation of chromosomal microarray analysis: summary of 2513 postnatal cases. PLoS One 2007;2(3):e327.

24. Edelmann L, Hirschhorn K. Clinical utility of array CGH for the detection of chromosomal imbalances associated with mental retardation and multiple congenital anomalies. Ann N Y Acad Sci 2009;1151:157–66.

25. Simovich MJ, Yatsenko SA, Kang SH, et al. Prenatal diagnosis of a 9q34.3 microdeletion by array-CGH in a fetus with an apparently balanced translocation. Prenat Diagn 2007;27(12):1112–7.

26. Rickman L, Fiegler H, Shaw-Smith C, et al. Prenatal detection of unbalanced chromosomal rearrangements by array CGH. J Med Genet 2006;43(4):353–61.

27. Larrabee PB, Johnson KL, Pestova E, et al. Microarray analysis of cell-free fetal DNA in amniotic fluid: a prenatal molecular karyotype. Am J Hum Genet 2004; 75(3):485–91.

28. Sahoo T, Cheung SW, Ward P, et al. Prenatal diagnosis of chromosomal abnormalities using array-based comparative genomic hybridization. Genet Med 2006;8(11):719–27.

29. Shaffer LG, Coppinger J, Alliman S, et al. Comparison of microarray-based detection rates for cytogenetic abnormalities in prenatal and neonatal specimens. Prenat Diagn 2008;28(9):789–95.

30. Van den Veyver IB, Patel A, Shaw CA, et al. Clinical use of array comparative genomic hybridization (aCGH) for prenatal diagnosis in 300 cases. Prenat Diagn 2009;29(1):29–39.

31. Coppinger J, Alliman S, Lamb AN, et al. Whole-genome microarray analysis in prenatal specimens identifies clinically significant chromosome alterations without increase in results of unclear significance compared to targeted microarray. Prenat Diagn 2009;29(12):1156–66.

32. Liehr T, Claussen U, Starke H. Small supernumerary marker chromosomes (sSMC) in humans. Cytogenet Genome Res 2004;107(1–2):55–67.

33. Choe J, Kang JK, Bae CJ, et al. Identification of origin of unknown derivative chromosomes by array-based comparative genomic hybridization using pre- and postnatal clinical samples. J Hum Genet 2007;52(11):934–42.
34. Ballif BC, Hornor SA, Sulpizio SG, et al. Development of a high-density pericentromeric region BAC clone set for the detection and characterization of small supernumerary marker chromosomes by array CGH. Genet Med 2007;9(3): 150–62.
35. Ballif BC, Rorem EA, Sundin K, et al. Detection of low-level mosaicism by array CGH in routine diagnostic specimens. Am J Med Genet A 2006;140(24):2757–67.
36. Gruchy N, Lebrun M, Herlicoviez M, et al. Supernumerary marker chromosomes management in prenatal diagnosis. Am J Med Genet A 2008;146(21):2770–6.
37. Youssoufian H, Pyeritz RE. Mechanisms and consequences of somatic mosaicism in humans. Nat Rev Genet 2002;3(10):748–58.
38. Hahnemann JM, Vejerslev LO. Accuracy of cytogenetic findings on chorionic villus sampling (CVS)—diagnostic consequences of CVS mosaicism and nonmosaic discrepancy in centres contributing to EUCROMIC 1986–1992. Prenat Diagn 1997;17(9):801–20.
39. Ledbetter DH, Zachary JM, Simpson JL, et al. Cytogenetic results from the U.S. Collaborative Study on CVS. Prenat Diagn 1992;12(5):317–45.
40. Bi W, Breman AM, Venable SF, et al. Rapid prenatal diagnosis using uncultured amniocytes and oligonucleotide array CGH. Prenat Diagn 2008;28(10):943–9.
41. Schaeffer AJ, Chung J, Heretis K, et al. Comparative genomic hybridization-array analysis enhances the detection of aneuploidies and submicroscopic imbalances in spontaneous miscarriages. Am J Hum Genet 2004;74(6):1168–74.
42. Benkhalifa M, Kasakyan S, Clement P, et al. Array comparative genomic hybridization profiling of first-trimester spontaneous abortions that fail to grow in vitro. Prenat Diagn 2005;25(10):894–900.
43. Shimokawa O, Harada N, Miyake N, et al. Array comparative genomic hybridization analysis in first-trimester spontaneous abortions with 'normal' karyotypes. Am J Med Genet A 2006;140(18):1931–5.
44. Menten B, Swerts K, Delle Chiaie B, et al. Array comparative genomic hybridization and flow cytometry analysis of spontaneous abortions and mors in utero samples. BMC Med Genet 2009;10:89.
45. Rajcan-Separovic E, Qiao Y, Tyson C, et al. Genomic changes detected by array CGH in human embryos with developmental defects. Mol Hum Reprod 2009; 16(2):125–34.
46. Darilek S, Ward P, Pursley A, et al. Pre- and postnatal genetic testing by array-comparative genomic hybridization: genetic counseling perspectives. Genet Med 2008;10(1):13–8.
47. Ogilvie CM, Yaron Y, Beaudet AL. Current controversies in prenatal diagnosis 3: for prenatal diagnosis, should we offer less or more than metaphase karyotyping? Prenat Diagn 2009;29(1):11–4.
48. Sapp JC, Hull SC, Duffer S, et al. Ambivalence toward undergoing invasive prenatal testing: an exploration of its origins. Prenat Diagn 2010;30(1):77–82.
49. ACOG Committee Opinion No. 446: array comparative genomic hybridization in prenatal diagnosis. Obstet Gynecol 2009;114(5):1161–3.

Screening, Testing, or Personalized Medicine: Where do Inherited Thrombophilias Fit Best?

Peggy Walker, MS[a], Anthony R. Gregg, MD[a,b],*

KEYWORDS

• Thrombophilia • Genetic screening • Pregnancy
• Adverse pregnancy outcomes • Factor V Leiden
• Prothrombin G20210A

Screening during pregnancy for conditions that affect a woman's health is not an unusual concept. Recommendations that advocate for gestational diabetes screening using a 1-hour glucose challenge and tuberculosis screening using the tuberculin skin test are widely followed.[1] However, there are no widely accepted practice recommendations for predisposition genetic screening of a maternal medical condition that can affect the fetus, health of a woman, and her relatives. This article focuses on the identification of those with inherited thrombophilias and the implications for pregnancy, addressing the question "Is screening appropriate for inherited thrombophilias?"

THE SCREENING PARADIGM

Concepts that must be distinguished include differentiating between screening and diagnostic testing. Population-based screening and diagnostic testing for mendelian-inherited conditions is different from predisposition screening for multifactorial or complex conditions (ie, conditions in which inherited disease-causing genes and

Funding: None.
[a] Division of Clinical Genetics and Molecular Medicine, Department of Obstetrics and Gynecology, University of South Carolina School of Medicine, Two Medical Park, Suite 103, Columbia, SC 29203, USA
[b] Division of Maternal Fetal Medicine, Department of Obstetrics and Gynecology, University of South Carolina School of Medicine, Two Medical Park, Suite 208, Columbia, SC 29203, USA
* Corresponding author. Division of Maternal-Fetal Medicine, Department of Obstetrics and Gynecology, University of South Carolina School of Medicine, Two Medical Park, Suite 208, Columbia, SC 29203.
E-mail address: anthony.gregg@uscmed.sc.edu

Obstet Gynecol Clin N Am 37 (2010) 87–107
doi:10.1016/j.ogc.2010.02.018
0889-8545/10/$ – see front matter © 2010 Elsevier Inc. All rights reserved.

environmental exposures interact to determine disease expression). Before considering these differences, the framework on which public health screening initiatives are undertaken is identified.

In 1968 Wilson and Jungner[2] established specific criteria for public health screening initiatives that would ideally be fulfilled before implementing screening programs. These criteria include the following:

1. The condition being screened for should be an important health problem.
2. The natural history of the condition should be well understood.
3. There should be a detectable early stage.
4. Treatment at an early stage should be of more benefit than at a later stage.
5. A suitable test should be devised for the early stage.
6. The test should be acceptable.
7. Intervals for repeating the test should be determined.
8. Adequate health service provision should be made for the extra clinical workload that results from screening.
9. The risks, physical and psychological, should be less than the benefits.
10. The costs should be balanced against the benefits.

The criteria have been applied across multiple disciplines of medicine[3] and continue to be considered by some as the gold standard for screening initiatives.[4] In 1975 the National Academy of Sciences (NAS) put forth similar screening criteria directed specifically at genetic disease screening.[5] This report included general, organizational, educational, legal, and research recommendations. The general recommendations are similar to those of Wilson and Jungner, but with a clear genetic screening perspective:

"Genetic screening when performed under controlled conditions is an appropriate form of medical care when the following criteria are met:

1. There is evidence of substantial public benefit and acceptance, including acceptance by medical practitioners.
2. Its feasibility has been investigated, and it has been found that benefits outweigh costs, appropriate public education can be performed, test methods are satisfactory, laboratory facilities are available, and resources exist to deal with counseling, follow-up, and other consequences of testing.
3. An investigative pretest of the program has shown that costs are acceptable, education is effective, informed consent is feasible, aims of the program with regard to the size of the sample to be screened, the age of the screenees, and the setting in which the testing is to be done have been defined, laboratory facilities have been shown to fulfill requirements for quality control, techniques for communicating results are workable, qualified and effective counselors are available in sufficient number, and adequate provision for effective services has been made.
4. The means are available to evaluate the effectiveness and success of each step in the process."

Although meeting most or all of these published criteria may justify screening for certain conditions, this does not mean that one should or must screen every condition that meets the criteria. Inherited thrombophilia screening is evaluated later in the context of criteria set forth by Wilson and Jungner as well as the NAS.

Screening programs usually start by focusing on at-risk subpopulations for conditions that satisfy Wilson and Jungner criteria 1 to 4. For mendelian disorders individuals within the at-risk subpopulation who are asymptomatic submit to a test that has satisfied the minimum criteria set forth by criteria 5 to 7. Most often, screening tests are not diagnostic tests; that is to say, a measureable false-positive and false-negative rate is associated with each screening test. Follow-up of a positive screening test results in the application of a diagnostic test. Diagnostic tests are often invasive and are typically more costly than screening tests. Positive diagnostic tests are intended to lead to treatments or increased surveillance. Obstetrician gynecologists are familiar with these concepts even when applied to complex diseases. The criteria of Wilson and Jungner applied to breast cancer screening illustrate these principles. A noninvasive screening test, mammography, is applied to an at-risk subpopulation (eg, based on gender and age). These individuals might be women aged 40 years, or persons with increased risk factors based on personal history or family history. Mammography is widely accepted, is suitable (noninvasive), and is performed at intervals that have been widely agreed on. Positive or suspicious tests are followed up using approaches that allow tissue to be studied directly (eg, invasive biopsy for diagnosis). Early stage diagnoses yield survival advantages. Breast cancer is a public health problem and its natural course has been well delineated.

Diagnostic testing schemes rely on specific criteria although not previously named. Entry is by way of any of 3 routes: (1) a positive screening test as described in the previous paragraph for breast cancer; (2) because family history suggests an increased risk; and (3) through patient-specific symptoms or signs of disease. For example, when a heritable condition affects first-degree relatives the term screening may not be the most appropriate. Colonoscopy and liberal use of endoscopic biopsy performed on a patient whose sibling or parent has hereditary nonpolyposis colon cancer is approached with a different medical mindset from colonoscopy starting at age 50 years performed for screening purposes in a family with no history of colorectal cancer. Also, a tuberculin skin test applied to a patient positive for the human immunodeficiency virus with a cough and an infiltrate on chest radiograph is not intended as a screening procedure. Rather, the intended purpose is in the diagnostic schema. Screening tests and screening procedures can be used as initial tests in establishing diagnoses.

GENETIC PRINCIPLES

Screening for genetic predisposition to disease with molecular approaches introduces new and unique concepts to the screening paradigm. The term carrier refers to persons who are asymptomatic and not at risk for the disease condition of interest (eg, cystic fibrosis carrier or spinal muscular atrophy carrier), but can pass the disease or propensity for the disease to their offspring. The term carrier is not appropriate for most of the common inherited thrombophilias, because most of the known thrombophilia disease-causing genetic mutations are dominant (**Table 1**). Carrier screening is performed when a family history does not exist. Testing is indicated when a family history can be documented. Thrombophilia testing may include either specific protein function studies (eg, antithrombin III activity testing), measurement of a serum-specific analyte (fasting homocysteine), or DNA analysis for 1 or more mutations in a specific gene known to be associated with the condition. Although DNA testing in this context might include an identical molecular approach as used in a population-based screening paradigm, it might also require that family-specific mutations be searched for that are not in the standard screening panel. Alternatively, this approach might require sequencing an entire gene for mutation identification.

Different populations can have varying frequencies of disease-causing mutations due to the founder effect. The founder effect results when a small subpopulation separates from an original population (usually hundreds of years earlier). If 1 individual of the subpopulation has a rare disease-causing mutation, then its frequency increases

Table 1
Characteristics of proteins and genes associated with key thrombophilia risk factors

Protein	Gene	Chromosome Location	Number of Exons (Gene Size in kb)	Thrombophilia-Specific Mutations	Inheritance Pattern	OMIM Reference	Testing Method[a]
Factor V	*F5*	1q23	25 (81)	R506Q (Factor V Leiden)	Dominant	*612309	DNA analysis
Prothrombin	*F2*	11p11-q12	14 (22)	G20210A	Dominant	+176930	DNA analysis
MTHFR	*MTHFR*	1p36.3	11 (22)	C677T/C677T C677T/A1298C	Recessive	*607093	DNA analysis
Antithrombin III	*SERPINC1*	1q23-q25	7 (15)	Rare variants	Dominant	*107300	Protein activity level
Protein C	*PROC*	2q13-q14	9 (12)	Rare variants	Dominant	#176860	Protein activity level
Protein S	*PROS1*	3q11.2	15 (111)	Rare variants	Dominant	#176880	Protein activity level

Abbreviations: MTHFR, methylenetetrahydrofolate reductase; ONIM, online Mendelian inheritance in man.
[a] Testing methods are the most definitive for identifying an inherited thrombophilia.

as that subpopulation expands.[6] The original population and the subpopulation can have varying incidence of the disease as a result of different disease-causing mutations. A well-known example of variation in the frequency of dominant BRCA1/2 disease-causing mutations has been documented in women of northern European ancestry (1 in 800 risk) compared with those of Ashkenazi Jewish descent, who have a 1 in 40 risk of carrying 1 of the 3 most common founder mutations (187delAG, 5385insC, and 6174delT) causing hereditary breast and ovarian cancer syndrome (see the article by Lee P. Shulman elsewhere in this issue for further exploration of this topic).

Residual risk refers to the risk of a patient carrying a diseased allele despite a negative molecular test. This concept is easiest to understand for the mendelian disorder cystic fibrosis. Non-Hispanic Whites whose carrier screen for cystic fibrosis is negative using the previously recommended 25-mutation panethnic panel have a 12% chance of being a carrier for an unidentified genetic mutation in the cystic fibrosis gene despite these results.[7] Testing patients for 1 or several mutations within a gene does not guarantee that the gene is free of all mutations. Thus, residual risk is a function of incomplete information and/or lack of knowledge (see the article by Jeffrey S. Dungan elsewhere in this issue for further exploration of this topic). Residual risk varies across ethnic groups. The same cystic fibrosis mutation panel and negative results in the Ashkenazi Jewish population lead to a residual risk of about 5%.

The terms mutation and polymorphism are often used interchangeably; however, subtle and often unappreciated differences exist. A mutation refers to an alteration in the DNA sequence of exons, introns, or regulatory regions of a gene. The alteration can be a disease-causing mutation, or it may not have clinical consequences. The terms polymorphism and rare variant are used to distinguish frequencies of DNA alterations. A polymorphism is defined as a change in a gene region that occurs with a frequency of greater than 1% in the general population. Polymorphisms may or may not cause/predispose to disease. Rare variants occur less commonly (ie, <1%) in the population and typically occur as a result of a spontaneous mutation in an individual within a specific family. Rare variants, or familial mutations, can then be inherited within family members but are usually not found commonly across the general population.[6] Taking these genetic principles into consideration, this article explores more deeply the relationship of thrombophilia identification and the Wilson and Jungner criteria.

THROMBOPHILIA BIOLOGY

Thrombophilia-related genes of interest can be divided into 3 groups based on the actions of the proteins they encode: procoagulants, natural anticoagulants, and fibrinolytic pathway proteins.[8] Procoagulant and natural anticoagulants have received the greatest attention; these will be our focus (see **Table 1**). Because coagulation, anticoagulation, and fibrinolysis are finely tuned pathways with many genetic factors, any testing or screening paradigm aimed at identifying thrombophilia results in residual risk, brought about by the number of unknown genes and mutations that could affect risk for thrombosis and/or by the limitations of the technology applied (ie, molecular laboratories test a variable number of genes for a variable number of mutations).

Procoagulants

F5 (Factor V)
The *F5* gene encodes the factor V protein, which when activated functions in the clotting cascade as part of the prothrombinase complex. This complex, which includes activated factor X, is a central focus within the clotting cascade and is responsible

for the conversion of prothrombin to thrombin (**Fig. 1**). Natural anticoagulant proteases inactivate the prothrombinase and tenase complexes. These natural anticoagulants include activated protein C (APC). There are 3 factor V cleavage sites prone to inactivation by protein C. The cleavage site at amino acid position 506 begins the degradation of factor V. The factor V Leiden mutation, a single nucleotide change (G1691A) that results in an amino acid substitution (R506Q), affects this site and is the most prevalent mutation of the *F5* gene. This cleavage site allows exposure of amino acids at positions 306 and 679 for further cleavage by APC. These 2 sites account for 70% and 30%, respectively, of the activity of factor V.[9] Mutations at key cleavage locations and others located throughout the *F5* gene result in resistance to APC inactivation.[10–14] *F5* mutations are inherited in an autosomal-dominant mendelian fashion. Heterozygotes with the mutation on 1 allele have a 7-fold increased risk of deep vein thrombosis (DVT), and homozygotes have a 42- to 79-fold increased risk of DVT.[15,16]

F2 (prothrombin)

The *F2* gene encodes clotting cascade factor II, also known as prothrombin. The prothrombinase complex cleaves this precursor protein to form thrombin (see **Fig. 1**). The subsequent formation of thrombin feeds back positively to promote the continued activation of factors V and VIII. The G20210A mutation at the noncoding 3′ end of the *F2* gene results in a gain of function mutation (enhanced transcriptional activity), promoting cleavage of factor II pre-mRNA, resulting in increased mRNA production. This mRNA increase of nearly 30% in heterozygous and 80% in homozygous model systems corresponds to increasing prothrombin activity and a proportionately increased risk for venous thromboembolic disease.[17,18] The *F2* gene is inherited in a dominant fashion.

MTHFR (methylenetetrahydrofolate reductase)

The *MTHFR* gene encodes the enzyme methylenetetrahydrofolate reductase (MTHFR). This enzyme plays a role in 1-carbon metabolism by converting 5,10-methylenetetrahydrofolate to 5-methyltetrahydrofolate. Folic acid is a precursor molecule

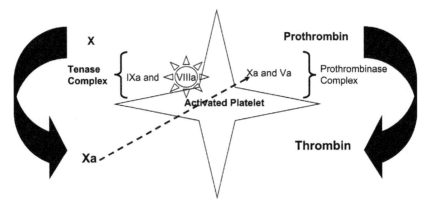

Fig. 1. Generation of thrombin through the prothrombinase complex. von Willebrand factor activates clotting factor VIII to VIIIa, which forms a complex with factor IXa to become the tenase complex. The tenase complex activates factor X to Xa, which then forms a complex with factor Va to create the prothrombinase complex. Prothrombin is converted to thrombin by the prothrombinase complex at the surface of activated platelets.

for the former. The latter is used as a cosubstrate for methylation of homocysteine to methionine (**Fig. 2**). The translated MTHFR protein consists of 2 functional regions, a 40-kDa catalytic and 37-kDa regulatory domain. Missense and nonsense mutations capable of altering enzyme activity have been described across the 22-kb gene.[19,20] Reduced enzyme activity leads to lower levels of 5-methyltetrahydrofolate and hence an increase in plasma homocysteine. The exact mechanism by which increased plasma homocysteine levels lead to enhanced blood clotting is unknown, but may be caused by an increase in reactive oxygen species that subsequently damage endothelial cells, leading to vascular smooth muscle proliferation, lipid peroxidation, and oxidation of low-density lipoproteins.[21] Mutations commonly tested for include a transition, C677T, and a transversion, A1298C. These genetic mutations are expressed as recessive alleles and 2 specific combinations (ie, C677T/C677T and C677T/A1298C) are believed to be clinically relevant. The C677T homozygous condition results in increased fasting plasma homocysteine levels under conditions of reduced folate

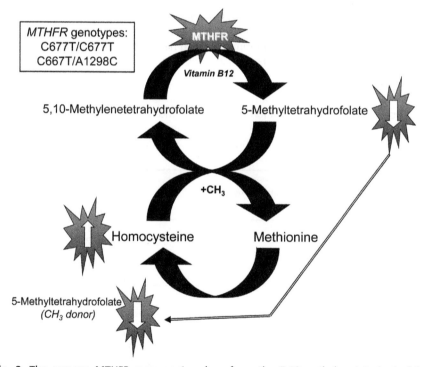

Fig. 2. The enzyme MTHFR removes 1 carbon from the 5,10-methylenetetrahydrofolate molecule to form 5-methyltetrahydrofolate. 5-Methyltetrahydrofolate acts as a methyl group donor for the remethylation of homocysteine to methionine. The C667T mutation in the *MTHFR* gene results in a thermolabile form of the enzyme, which decreases the availability of 5-methyltetrahydrofolate. Decreased cofactor for the conversion of homocysteine to methionine results in increased plasma homocysteine levels, which have been shown to increase procoagulant activity. Homozygous C667T/C667T and compound heterozygous C667T/A1298C genotypes have been reported to increase the predisposition to thrombophilia. (*Data from* Hanson NQ, Aras O, Yang F, et al. C677T and A1298C polymorphisms of the methylenetetrahydrofolate reductase gene: incidence and effect of combined genotypes on plasma fasting and post-methionine load homocysteine in vascular disease. Clin Chem 2001;47:661–6.)

stores.[22] Data point to increased plasma homocysteine levels in individuals with the C677T/A1298C genotype compared with those with a normal genotype, although the clinical relevance remains in question.[23] Clinicians often use fasting plasma homocysteine levels as an initial test to determine the need for DNA testing.

Natural Anticoagulants

SERPINC1 (antithrombin III)
SERPINC1 encodes antithrombin III, a serine protease that functions to inactivate coagulation pathway serine proteases factor Xa and thrombin.[24–26] Antithrombin also has inhibitory properties on several other clotting factors (eg, IXa, XIa, XIIa)[27,28] and a fibrinolytic pathway protein, plasmin.[29] Antithrombin activity is greatly improved through heparin binding.[30] This latter point emphasizes the primary mechanism of heparin in effecting anticoagulation. This gene has 7 exons and the genomic sequence spans more than 13 kb.[31] Family-specific mutations (rare variants) preclude DNA-based mutation analysis in the clinical setting except for rare circumstances. Therefore, functional assays are the primary method of testing for antithrombin III-associated thrombophilia. Antithrombin III functions as a dominant gene and inactivating mutations in this gene result in significant risk for venous thromboembolic events. Antithrombin III deficiency is not common among healthy people (**Table 2**); however, a 10-fold increase in prevalence is seen in select populations.[32]

PROC (protein C)
PROC encodes protein C, a vitamin K-dependent natural anticoagulant that when activated results in the inactivation of factors V and VIII. Protein C is activated by the thrombomodulin/thrombin complex, which binds to the endothelium, activating protein C through a cleavage mechanism. APC binds to protein S and results in

Table 2 Population frequency of thrombophilia risk factors	
Protein	**Population Frequency (%)**
Factor V[67]	White: 5.5 Hispanic: 2.2 African American: 1.2 European: 3–10 Asian: 0.5
Prothrombin[68,69]	White: 0.7–4.0 Mexican American: 1.1 African American: 0.3 European: 1.7–3 Italian: 4–6 Asian, Native American: rare
MTHFR[23]	United States: C667T heterozygous: 46 C667T homozygous: 12 A1298C heterozygous: 40 C667T/A1298C: 15–20
Antithrombin III[70]	Unselected population 0.02–0.20
Protein C[71]	Unselected population 0.3–0.5
Protein S[72]	Unselected population 0.2–0.4

inactivation of Va and VIIIa (**Fig. 3**). Like antithrombin III, sequence variation in protein C is extensive and inheritance is dominant. Diagnostic testing uses primarily activity assays rather than mutational analysis because of the occurrence of familial mutations (rare variants).

PROS1 (protein S)

Protein S is a vitamin K-dependent protein encoded by the *PROS1* gene and serves as a natural anticoagulant cofactor for APC (see **Fig. 3**). Protein S is also involved in protein interactions with procoagulation factors Va, VIIIa, and Xa.[33] Thus, protein S serves to modulate the procoagulant system in multiple ways. Deficiency of protein S leads to increased risk of thrombosis. Protein S circulates in the human plasma as free protein S and also bound to complement C4b-binding protein, which inactivates the anticoagulant properties of protein S. The balance between free and bound protein S affects propensity toward thrombosis. Pregnancy is known to decrease protein S activity. Functional and immunologic protein S levels are decreased during pregnancy.[34] Functional activity measurements of protein S are preferable to antigen concentration to identify those individuals with thrombophilia caused by protein S deficiency, as some patients may have adequate concentration of protein S but decreased functional activity. Samples for protein S activity should be drawn before the initiation of anticoagulation therapy (when establishing a diagnosis of protein S deficiency) because patients receiving oral anticoagulants (eg, warfarin) will have decreased functional activity of protein S and protein C. Similarly to antithrombin III and protein C, various unique familial DNA mutations of *PROS1* result in protein S deficiency with dominant expression.

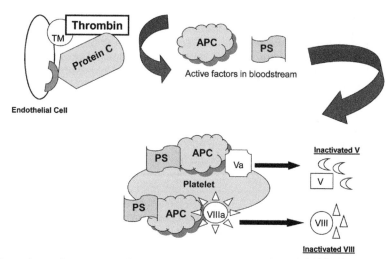

Fig. 3. Anticoagulant activity of protein C and protein S. Protein C binds to endothelial cells via the endothelial cell protein C receptor (EPCR). Thrombomodulin (TM) on the surface of endothelial cells acts as a cofactor with thrombin to activate protein C bound to EPCR. APC is released from the endothelial cell surface into the bloodstream. APC and protein S (PS) form a complex on the surface of activated platelets to degrade activated clotting factor Va and activated VIIIa, resulting in inhibition of the procoagulant system. (*Data from* Kottke-Marchant K, Comp P. Laboratory issues in diagnosing abnormalities of protein C, thrombomodulin, and endothelial cell protein C receptor. Arch Pathol Lab Med 2002;126:1337–48.)

PHENOTYPES AND CASE-CONTROL STUDIES

There is evidence that inherited thrombophilias affect the venous and arterial vasculature in a gene-specific way.[12] The maternal phenotype, venous thromboembolism (VTE), is most common. Adverse pregnancy outcomes (APOs) include intrauterine growth restriction (IUGR), severe preeclampsia, placental abruption, and stillbirth. These outcomes have been studied extensively for their association with inherited thrombophilias.

Virchow's triad (ie, stasis, hypercoagulable state, and trauma) is a reminder that pregnancy confers a risk for venous thromboembolic disease. The primary antecedents during pregnancy are the hypercoagulable state resulting from a unique hormonal milieu and physiologic changes of pregnancy, the increased venous stasis brought on by the gravid uterus and loss of vasomotor tone during anesthesia, and in some cases trauma related to surgical procedures. The magnitude of the VTE risk in unselected patients is about 4.29 (3.49–5.22, $P<.001$) during pregnancy (antepartum and postpartum periods) compared with nonpregnant patients.[35] Identification of a factor V Leiden mutation was associated with a 0.25% probability of venous thrombosis during pregnancy, compared with a baseline VTE risk of 0.03%. When the prothrombin gene mutation (G20210A) was identified, the risk was 0.5%. Antithrombin III deficiency and protein C deficiency were associated with a 0.4% and 0.1% risk, respectively. Risk was greatest when the factor V Leiden and prothrombin gene were identified in the same patient (4.6%).[36]

The composite prevalence of APO is 8%. IUGR and severe preeclampsia are the most common, at about 5% and 2%, respectively.[37] The earliest reports linking inherited thrombophilia with APO took advantage of case-control methods (**Fig. 4**). In a report by Kupferminc and colleagues,[38] the pregnancy outcomes of 110 patients with inherited thrombophilia were compared with patients without thrombophilia. Significant relationships were seen. van Pampus and colleagues[39] found no relationship between factor V Leiden and preeclampsia among 345 patients with severe preeclampsia and 67 controls. De Groot and colleagues[40] compared 163 matched cases and controls and found no association of preeclampsia with factor V Leiden or prothrombin G20210A genotype. Case-control studies of IUGR, stillbirth, and placental abruption also vary. In a study by Many and colleagues[41] that looked at specific inherited thrombophilias, 40 cases and 80 controls showed that several specific thrombophilias were associated with stillbirth after 27 weeks' gestation. Although Hefler and colleagues[42] concluded there was no association between inherited thrombophilias and stillbirth among 94 cases and 94 controls, they acknowledged their study was underpowered (15%–33%) and the number needed to achieve 80% power would have been 1200 to 3800 women per group. These investigators concluded that case-control studies of thrombophilia in pregnancy are not easily interpreted because they are underpowered. **Fig. 4** shows inconclusive results for a relationship between common inherited defects in the coagulation pathway and APO. There are limited data on the relationship of APO and natural anticoagulation defects, most likely because of the low frequency of these mutations in European populations (rare variants, see **Table 2**).

PREGNANCY, THROMBOPHILIA, AND COHORT STUDIES

A genetic screening approach to identify thrombophilias with the goal of averting APO can be recommended only if a relationship between thrombophilia and APO can be clearly shown. This relationship is difficult to prove because of the complex pathogenesis of thrombosis and the variable expressivity of APO (eg, preeclampsia phenotypes). To date, no study has addressed all possible pathways to thrombosis or genotypes known to be associated with thrombosis. No study has simultaneously

Adverse Pregnancy Outcomes: Case-Control Studies

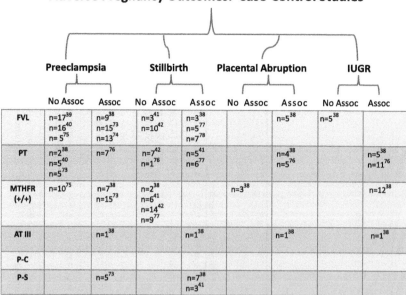

	Preeclampsia		Stillbirth		Placental Abruption		IUGR	
	No Assoc	Assoc	No Assoc	Assoc	No Assoc	Assoc	No Assoc	Assoc
FVL	n=17[39] n=16[40] n=5[75]	n=9[38] n=15[73] n=13[74]	n=3[41] n=10[42]	n=3[38] n=5[77] n=7[78]		n=5[38]	n=5[38]	
PT	n=2[38] n=5[40] n=5[73]	n=7[76]	n=7[42] n=1[76]	n=5[41] n=6[77]		n=4[38] n=5[76]		n=5[38] n=11[76]
MTHFR (+/+)	n=10[75]	n=7[38] n=15[73]	n=2[38] n=6[41] n=14[42] n=9[77]		n=3[38]			n=12[38]
AT III		n=1[38]		n=1[38]		n=1[38]		n=1[38]
P-C								
P-S		n=5[73]		n=7[38] n=3[41]				

Fig. 4. Reports of APOs from selected case-control studies. Assoc, association of statistical significance for increased risk of specific outcome; AT III, antithrombin III; FVL, factor V Leiden; MTHFR, methylene tetrahydrofolate reductase; n, number of cases with specific risk factor and possible association with specific APO; No assoc, lack of statistical significance of association between risk factor and outcome; P-C, protein C; P-S, protein S; PT, prothrombin gene. Publications reviewed are not intended to be a comprehensive review of all relevant literature on this topic, but rather to show conflicting results of several case-control studies.[38–42,73–78]

addressed procoagulant mutations, natural anticoagulant mutations, and fibrinolytic pathway abnormalities (eg, plasminogen activator inhibitor), all capable of influencing phenotypic expression.

Early in the evolution to the current evidence base, case-control (genetic association) studies dominated investigations (see **Fig. 4**). These studies yielded to meta-analyses with confirmatory results,[43–45] which were challenged by others who cited publication bias and sample size as causes of erroneous associations.[46] Cohort studies, prospective and with large numbers of patients, have also been explored (**Table 3**). These studies focus predominantly on factor V Leiden and the prothrombin gene mutation (G20210A) and avoid the problem of rare variants (eg, deficiencies of antithrombin III, protein S, and protein C). These studies vary with respect to primary outcome measures, number of genes interrogated, ethnic group studied, and statistical approaches used to draw conclusions. Despite these variations, some significant findings have been reported. In aggregate these studies suggest a relationship between factor V Leiden and stillbirth, preeclampsia, and placental abruption. Abstract summaries of these studies[47–51] along with corresponding editorials[52] place emphasis on statistically insignificant findings and ignore findings that reach significance.

FAMILY HISTORY AS A HELPFUL TOOL

The breast cancer screening paradigm (see article by Lee P. Shulman elsewhere in this issue for further exploration of this topic) has set a valuable precedent for the use of family history as an aid to determine which patients might benefit from thrombophilia

Table 3
Selected cohort studies of inherited thrombophilia and pregnancy outcome

Author Year (References)	Gene/Mutation[a]	Primary Outcome	Study Group[b]	Patient Ethnicity	Number	Results
Said et al 2010[49]	F5/R506Q F2/G20210A MTHFR/C677T MTHFR/A1298C Thrombomodulin	Severe preeclampsia, SGA (<5%, <10%), abruption, stillbirth, neonatal death	Healthy Nulliparous Family Hx (−) Personal Hx (−)	Unknown: 46% Northern European: 36%	1707	Composite outcome: F2 (+) = OR: 3.6 (1.2–10.6), $P = .04$ MTHFR (A1298C/A1298C) OR: 0.3 (0.1–.9), $P = .03$ F5 (+), Stillbirth OR: 8.9 (1.6–48.9) F2 (+), Abruption OR 12.2 (2.5–60.4), $P = .0$ MTHFR, A1298C/wt and A1298C/ A1298C genotypes protect against SGA
Silver et al 2010[51]	F2/G20210A	Preeclampsia, SGA (<5%, <10%), abruption, stillbirth	Unselected Family Hx (−)	Not reported	4167	APOs were not associated with F2 genotype
Coppens et al 2007[50]	F5/R506Q F2/G20210A	Successful pregnancy outcome after early or late unexplained loss	Family Hx (+) or increased FVIII, homocysteine, and VTE	Northern European[b]	993	Successful outcome after prior pregnancy loss is not related to F5 or F2 genotype

Study	Polymorphism	Outcomes	Selection	Race	N	Results
Kocher et al 2007[48]	F5/R506Q F2/G20210A	Miscarriage, preeclampsia, SGA (<5%, <10%), abruption, stillbirth, PTD	Selected (no Hx APA, lupus or LAC)	W = 73%	4872	Data all patients F5 (+): Stillbirth: OR, 4.3 (1.8–10.2), P = .001 Data for W F5 (+): Stillbirth: OR, 11.6 (1.9–69.4), P = .007 Preterm delivery: OR, 3.2 (1.1–9.3), P = .04
Dizon-Townsend et al 2005[47]	F5/R506Q	VTE (preeclampsia, SGA (<5%, <10%), abruption, stillbirth	Unselected Personal Hx (–)	F5 (+): W 69%, H 19%, AA 10% F5 (–): W 30%, H 32%, AA 36%	4885	VTE not associated with genotype F5 (+) and preeclampsia AA, RR: 3.9 (1.3–9.9), P = .04 H, RR: 4.8 (1.6–12.8), P = .3

Abbreviations: AA, African American; APA, antiphospholipid antibodies; APC resistance is a surrogate test for factor V mutation study; H, Hispanic; LAC, lupus anticoagulants; OR, odds ratio; PTD, preterm delivery; RR, relative risk; SGA, small for gestational age; W, white; wt, wild type.
[a] Amino acid or nucleotide substitution.
[b] In some cases inferred from research institution Hx (–), no history of venous thrombophilia or antiphospholipid syndrome.

screening. Similarities between the breast cancer predisposition screening paradigm and thrombophilia predisposition screening include multifactorial condition (ie, interactions between environmental and genetic factors), ethnic specific risk, and a residual risk persisting after negative results of mutation testing. Investigators have suggested that selecting those individuals who might benefit most from breast cancer predisposition genetic screening can be guided by family history. In 1 such approach, 3-generation pedigrees are scored as average risk (ie, population risk), moderate risk, or high risk. Patients whose family history is determined to be high risk are recommended for referral to a genetic professional for counseling surrounding predisposition genetic testing for breast cancer.[53]

Various studies have reported on the possible usefulness of assessing an individual's family history to estimate the level of risk for thrombophilia. One study that incorporated family history of VTE to address VTE risk among oral contraceptive users found a low sensitivity and a low positive predictive value.[54] A population-based, case-control study by Bezemer and colleagues[55] showed that a positive family history increased the risk of a first VTE by about 2-fold. However, association between family history and genetic risk factors was low. These investigators concluded that family history of VTE is a risk indicator because it represents increased susceptibility as a result of environmental and genetic susceptibility factors. The Inherited Pregnancy Loss Working Group of the National Society of Genetic Counselors published recommendations in 2005[56] that personal and family history of thrombophilia or identified genetic mutations be included in the 3-generation family history of an individual with recurrent pregnancy losses. Silver and Warren[57] recommended that genetic testing for possible causes of thrombophilia be performed in patients with personal or family history of thrombosis. These investigators also stated that thrombophilia testing should be considered for patients with family history of thrombosis or pregnancy history of unexplained fetal death, severe early onset preeclampsia, severe IUGR, or severe placental insufficiency. Varga[58] suggested that a 3- to 4-generation family history with questions targeted toward thrombophilia and verification by medical records when possible should be included when assessing the likelihood of thrombophilia in a patient within a genetic counseling session. Although most investigators recommend that patients with a personal or family history of thrombophilia be referred to a genetic counselor or other genetic professional, there are still inadequate data on how family history can guide predisposition screening for thrombophilia among pregnant patients at risk for VTE or APO.

PERSONALIZED MEDICINE

With today's genomic and genetic testing capabilities, personalized medicine is becoming, in some instances, a reality. In breast cancer diagnosis and treatment, oncologists can now determine if the malignant tumor tissue shows overamplification of a specific gene, HER2/neu, leading to overexpression of the HER2 receptor protein in about 30% of invasive breast cancers.[59] If this genetic alteration is identified, then the patient is a candidate for trastuzumab (Herceptin) therapy, which specifically targets tumor cells overexpressing the HER2 receptor. As we apply family history and the mendelian rules of inheritance to assess the possible risk of specific conditions, we are providing personalized risk information. When we act on that information, we are providing patients with personalized medicine. In similar ways that we have personalized risk assessment and treatment of women with inherited causes of breast cancer, we believe that pregnant women with suspected inherited susceptibility to thrombophilia can benefit from a personalized medicine approach. Personal medical and pregnancy history, 3-generation family history, and appropriate screening of targeted individuals for selective thrombophilia testing can lead to personalized management of pregnancies in women with thrombophilia, in the hope of improved outcomes.

THE POSITION OF PROFESSIONAL ORGANIZATIONS

The American College of Medical Genetics consensus statement on factor V Leiden mutation testing focused on 8 relevant questions.[60] Among these questions was who should be tested for this mutation. The statement concluded that "there is a growing consensus that testing should be performed in at least the following circumstances" relevant to pregnant women

- Venous thrombosis in pregnant women or women taking oral contraceptives
- Relatives of individuals less than 50 years old with venous thrombosis

The statement noted that testing may also be considered for the following persons

- Relatives of individuals known to have factor V Leiden ("Knowledge that they have factor V Leiden may influence management of pregnancy and may be a factor in decision-making regarding oral contraceptive use")
- Women with recurrent pregnancy loss or unexplained severe preeclampsia, placental abruption, intrauterine fetal growth retardation, or stillbirth ("Knowledge of factor V Leiden carrier status may influence management of future pregnancies").

This working group also stated that the "random screening of the general population for factor V Leiden is not recommended."

The College of American Pathologists Consensus Conference (XXXVI) convened in 2001 to discuss laboratory testing for thrombophilia based on medical literature and expert opinions.[61] Overall, they concluded that factor V Leiden mutation, prothrombin mutation G20210A, functional protein C, functional protein S, and functional antithrombin III assays are appropriate for specific patients[62–66] and recommended testing for thrombophilia in individuals with the following medical history or conditions

- A history of recurrent VTE
- less than 50 years old with VTE
- Unprovoked VTE at any age (however, testing for protein C, protein S, or antithrombin deficiency may be of lower diagnostic yield if patient with first lifetime VTE after age 50 years)
- VTE at unusual sites
- Patients with VTE with a family history of VTE
- VTE secondary to pregnancy, oral contraceptive use, or hormone replacement therapy.

The Consensus Conference specifically recommended thrombophilia testing for the following 3 classes of women patients

- Women with VTE during pregnancy or in the postpartum period
- Women with pregnancy loss that is either recurrent or late in the pregnancy (in the second or third trimester)
- Women who experience VTE as cerebral venous thrombosis during oral contraceptive intake or hormone replacement therapy.

The Conference stated that thrombophilia testing women with other gestational complications is controversial and noted that results of protein S testing during pregnancy or the postpartum period should be interpreted with caution because of physiologic changes.

The American College of Obstetricians and Gynecologists is currently silent on predisposition genetic screening for thrombophilia.

PUBLIC HEALTH SCREENING CRITERIA AND INHERITED THROMBOPHILIA

All criteria posited by Wilson and Jungner[2] cannot be adequately addressed in inherited thrombophilias.

1. Thrombophilia is an important health problem.
2. The natural history of thrombophilia is not yet completely understood, with additional pathways, genes, and mutations expected to be further elucidated.
3. The criteria, "there should be a detectable early stage," does not apply to thrombophilia-related phenotypes (eg, stroke, heart attack, DVT, and pulmonary embolism).
4. With no detectable early stage, early treatment benefits are not applicable to this condition.
5. Noninvasive blood tests are available to measure the 6 known genetic factors that can predispose a patient to thrombophilia.
6. Current tests are acceptable and can be validated per standard laboratory requirements for specificity and sensitivity.
7. Interval testing is not applicable to genetic testing for thrombophilia.
8. Adequate workload provisions have not been made to address the increased demand for genetics counseling that would be required if thrombophilia screening were implemented.
9. The risks and benefits from implementing a screening program for thrombophilia are unknown.
10. Limited data are available for cost/benefit analysis.

Furthermore, the NAS criteria for genetic screening[5] are also not met:

1. We accept that identification of individuals with inherited thrombophilia can lead to individual health benefits and that the burden on health care providers to select appropriate patients for testing is not onerous. However, uncertainty remains about specific pregnancy outcomes that stem from thrombophilia-associated risk factors such that substantial benefit to public health remains unknown.
2. Although test methods are satisfactory and laboratory facilities are available, cost efficacy has not been established and counseling resources are not adequately addressed in practice or on paper.
3. An investigative pretest program for widespread genetic screening for thrombophilia has not been established.
4. An evaluative tool to monitor efficacy of such a screening program is not in place and has not been described.

SUMMARY

- Screening unselected reproductive-age women for thrombophilia is inconsistent with the Wilson and Jungner screening paradigm and does not meet the criteria for genetic screening proposed by the NAS.

- A personalized medicine approach is most appropriate in assessing a pregnant patient's risk for thrombophilia.
- Because of the multifactorial nature of thrombophilia phenotypes, residual risk for inherited thrombophilia must be considered even after negative test results. There are no data to guide the physician's discussion with patients regarding the magnitude of this risk.
- Data from large cohort studies suggest that specific thrombophilia mutations (eg, factor V Leiden and prothrombin G20210A) may predispose pregnant women to APOs.
- Data are limited with respect to the effect of family history and how this can enhance clinical usefulness of tests for inherited thrombophilia.

ACKNOWLEDGMENTS

The authors acknowledge the expert technical assistance of Amy Anderson and Ericka Weaver in the preparation of this manuscript.

REFERENCES

1. Perinatal infections. In: Lockwood CJ, Lemons JA, Riley LE, et al, editors. Guidelines for perinatal care. 6th edition. Washington, DC: The American Academy of Pediatrics and the American College of Obstetricians and Gynecologists; 2007. p. 335–9.
2. Wilson JM, Jungner G. Principles and practice of screening for disease. Geneva: World Health Organization; 1968.
3. Newborn screening: toward a uniform screening panel and system. Genet Med 2006;8(Suppl 1):1S–252S.
4. Andermann A, Blancquaert I, Beauchamp S, et al. Revisiting Wilson and Jungner in the genomic age: a review of screening criteria over the past 40 years. Bull World Health Organ 2008;86:317–9.
5. Simopoulos AP. Genetic screening: programs, principles, and research–thirty years later. Reviewing the recommendations of the Committee for the Study of Inborn Errors of Metabolism (SIEM). Public Health Genomics 2009;12:105–11.
6. Nussbaum RL, McInnes RR, Huntington FW. Genetic variation in individuals and populations: mutations and polymorphism. Thompson and Thompson Genetics in Medicine. 7th edition. Philadelphia: Saunders Elsevier; 2007. p. 201–2, 183.
7. ACOG Committee on Genetics. Update on carrier screening for cystic fibrosis. Washington, DC: American College of Obstetricians and Gynecologists; 2005.
8. Dahlback B. Advances in understanding pathogenic mechanisms of thrombophilic disorders. Blood 2008;112:19–27.
9. Kalafatis M, Bertina RM, Rand MD, et al. Characterization of the molecular defect in factor VR506Q. J Biol Chem 1995;270:4053–7.
10. Lunghi B, Castoldi E, Mingozzi F, et al. A novel factor V null mutation detected in a thrombophilic patient with pseudo-homozygous APC resistance and in an asymptomatic unrelated subject. Blood 1998;92:1463–4.
11. Williamson D, Brown K, Luddington R, et al. Factor V Cambridge: a new mutation (Arg306→Thr) associated with resistance to activated protein C. Blood 1998;91:1140–4.
12. Castoldi E, Simioni P, Kalafatis M, et al. Combinations of 4 mutations (FV R506Q, FV H1299R, FV Y1702C, PT 20210G/A) affecting the prothrombinase complex in a thrombophilic family. Blood 2000;96:1443–8.

13. Brugge JM, Simioni P, Bernardi F, et al. Expression of the normal factor V allele modulates the APC resistance phenotype in heterozygous carriers of the factor V Leiden mutation. J Thromb Haemost 2005;3:2695–702.

14. Lunghi B, Scanavini D, Castoldi E, et al. The factor V Glu1608Lys mutation is recurrent in familial thrombophilia. J Thromb Haemost 2005;3:2032–8.

15. Rosendaal FR, Koster T, Vandenbroucke JP, et al. High risk of thrombosis in patients homozygous for factor V Leiden (activated protein C resistance). Blood 1995;85:1504–8.

16. Hainaut P, Azerad MA, Lehmann E, et al. Prevalence of activated protein C resistance and analysis of clinical profile in thromboembolic patients. A Belgian prospective study. J Intern Med 1997;241:427–33.

17. Poort SR, Rosendaal FR, Reitsma PH, et al. A common genetic variation in the 3'-untranslated region of the prothrombin gene is associated with elevated plasma prothrombin levels and an increase in venous thrombosis. Blood 1996; 88:3698–703.

18. Gehring NH, Frede U, Neu-Yilik G, et al. Increased efficiency of mRNA 3' end formation: a new genetic mechanism contributing to hereditary thrombophilia. Nat Genet 2001;28:389–92.

19. Yano H, Nakaso K, Yasui K, et al. Mutations of the MTHFR gene (428C>T and [458G>T+459C>T]) markedly decrease MTHFR enzyme activity. Neurogenetics 2004;5:135–40.

20. Leclerc D, Sibani S, Rozen R. Molecular biology of methylenetetrahydrofolate reductase (MTHFR) and overview of mutations/polymorphisms. In: Ueland M, Rozen R, editors. MTHFR polymorphisms and disease. Austin (TX): Landes Bioscience; 2005. Available at: http://www.ncbi.nlm.nih.gov/bookshelf/br.fcgi?book= eurekah&part=A52348. Accessed January 29, 2010.

21. Welch GN, Loscalzo J. Homocysteine and atherothrombosis. N Engl J Med 1998; 338:1042–50.

22. Jacques PF, Bostom AG, Williams RR, et al. Relation between folate status, a common mutation in methylenetetrahydrofolate reductase, and plasma homocysteine concentrations. Circulation 1996;93:7–9.

23. Hanson NQ, Aras O, Yang F, et al. C677T and A1298C polymorphisms of the methylenetetrahydrofolate reductase gene: incidence and effect of combined genotypes on plasma fasting and post-methionine load homocysteine in vascular disease. Clin Chem 2001;47:661–6.

24. Rosenberg RD, Damus PS. The purification and mechanism of action of human antithrombin-heparin cofactor. J Biol Chem 1973;248:6490–505.

25. Buchanan MR, Boneu B, Ofosu F, et al. The relative importance of thrombin inhibition and factor Xa inhibition to the antithrombotic effects of heparin. Blood 1985; 65:198–201.

26. Kurachi K, Fujikawa K, Schmer G, et al. Inhibition of bovine factor IXa and factor Xabeta by antithrombin III. Biochemistry 1976;15:373–7.

27. Scott CF, Colman RW. Factors influencing the acceleration of human factor XIa inactivation by antithrombin III. Blood 1989;73:1873–9.

28. Stead N, Kaplan AP, Rosenberg RD. Inhibition of activated factor XII by antithrombin-heparin cofactor. J Biol Chem 1976;251:6481–8.

29. Highsmith RF, Rosenberg RD. The inhibition of human plasmin by human antithrombin-heparin cofactor. J Biol Chem 1974;249:4335–8.

30. Jin L, Abrahams JP, Skinner R, et al. The anticoagulant activation of antithrombin by heparin. Proc Natl Acad Sci U S A 1997;94:14683–8.

31. Olds RJ, Lane DA, Chowdhury V, et al. Complete nucleotide sequence of the antithrombin gene: evidence for homologous recombination causing thrombophilia. Biochemistry 1993;32:4216–24.
32. Heijboer H, Brandjes DP, Buller HR, et al. Deficiencies of coagulation-inhibiting and fibrinolytic proteins in outpatients with deep-vein thrombosis. N Engl J Med 1990;323:1512–6.
33. Rigby AC, Grant MA. Protein S: a conduit between anticoagulation and inflammation. Crit Care Med 2004;32:S336–41.
34. Comp PC, Thurnau GR, Welsh J, et al. Functional and immunologic protein S levels are decreased during pregnancy. Blood 1986;68:881–5.
35. Heit JA, Kobbervig CE, James AH, et al. Trends in the incidence of venous thromboembolism during pregnancy or postpartum: a 30-year population-based study. Ann Intern Med 2005;143:697–706.
36. Gerhardt A, Scharf RE, Beckmann MW, et al. Prothrombin and factor V mutations in women with a history of thrombosis during pregnancy and the puerperium. N Engl J Med 2000;342:374–80.
37. Paidas MJ, Ku DH, Arkel YS. Screening and management of inherited thrombophilias in the setting of adverse pregnancy outcome. Clin Perinatol 2004;31: 783–805, vii.
38. Kupferminc MJ, Eldor A, Steinman N, et al. Increased frequency of genetic thrombophilia in women with complications of pregnancy. N Engl J Med 1999;340: 9–13.
39. van Pampus MG, Dekker GA, Wolf H, et al. High prevalence of hemostatic abnormalities in women with a history of severe preeclampsia. Am J Obstet Gynecol 1999;180:1146–50.
40. De Groot CJ, Bloemenkamp KW, Duvekot EJ, et al. Preeclampsia and genetic risk factors for thrombosis: a case-control study. Am J Obstet Gynecol 1999;181: 975–80.
41. Many A, Elad R, Yaron Y, et al. Third-trimester unexplained intrauterine fetal death is associated with inherited thrombophilia. Obstet Gynecol 2002;99:684–7.
42. Hefler L, Jirecek S, Heim K, et al. Genetic polymorphisms associated with thrombophilia and vascular disease in women with unexplained late intrauterine fetal death: a multicenter study. J Soc Gynecol Investig 2004;11:42–4.
43. Howley HE, Walker M, Rodger MA. A systematic review of the association between factor V Leiden or prothrombin gene variant and intrauterine growth restriction. Am J Obstet Gynecol 2005;192:694–708.
44. Alfirevic Z, Roberts D, Martlew V. How strong is the association between maternal thrombophilia and adverse pregnancy outcome? A systematic review. Eur J Obstet Gynecol Reprod Biol 2002;101:6–14.
45. Robertson L, Wu O, Langhorne P, et al. Thrombophilia in pregnancy: a systematic review. Br J Haematol 2006;132:171–96.
46. Facco F, You W, Grobman W. Genetic thrombophilias and intrauterine growth restriction: a meta-analysis. Obstet Gynecol 2009;113:1206–16.
47. Dizon-Townson D, Miller C, Sibai B, et al. The relationship of the factor V Leiden mutation and pregnancy outcomes for mother and fetus. Obstet Gynecol 2005; 106:517–24.
48. Kocher O, Cirovic C, Malynn E, et al. Obstetric complications in patients with hereditary thrombophilia identified using the LCx microparticle enzyme immunoassay: a controlled study of 5,000 patients. Am J Clin Pathol 2007;127:68–75.
49. Said JM, Higgins JR, Moses EK, et al. Inherited thrombophilia polymorphisms and pregnancy outcomes in nulliparous women. Obstet Gynecol 2010;115:5–13.

50. Coppens M, van Mourik JA, Eckmann CM, et al. Current practise of testing for inherited thrombophilia. J Thromb Haemost 2007;5:1979–81.
51. Silver RM, Zhao Y, Spong CY, et al. Prothrombin gene G20210A mutation and obstetric complications. Obstet Gynecol 2010;115:14–20.
52. Branch DW. The truth about inherited thrombophilias and pregnancy. Obstet Gynecol 2010;115:2–4.
53. U.S. Preventive Services Task Force. Genetic risk assessment and BRCA mutation testing for breast and ovarian cancer susceptibility: recommendation statement. Ann Intern Med 2005;143:355–61.
54. Cosmi B, Legnani C, Bernardi F, et al. Role of family history in identifying women with thrombophilia and higher risk of venous thromboembolism during oral contraception. Arch Intern Med 2003;163:1105–9.
55. Bezemer ID, van der Meer FJ, Eikenboom JC, et al. The value of family history as a risk indicator for venous thrombosis. Arch Intern Med 2009;169:610–5.
56. Laurino MY, Bennett RL, Saraiya DS, et al. Genetic evaluation and counseling of couples with recurrent miscarriage: recommendations of the National Society of Genetic Counselors. J Genet Couns 2005;14:165–81.
57. Silver RM, Warren JE. Preconception counseling for women with thrombophilia. Clin Obstet Gynecol 2006;49:906–19.
58. Varga E. Inherited thrombophilia: key points for genetic counseling. J Genet Couns 2007;16:261–77.
59. Markman M. Breast cancer and HER2. eMedicine Specialties at Genomic Medicine at Oncology. 26 July 2009. Medscape. Available at: http://emedicine.medscape.com/article/1689966-overview. Accessed January 26, 2010.
60. Grody WW, Griffin JH, Taylor AK, et al. American College of Medical Genetics consensus statement on factor V Leiden mutation testing. Genet Med 2001;3:139–48.
61. Olson JD. College of American Pathologists Consensus Conference XXXVI: diagnostic issues in thrombophilia. Arch Pathol Lab Med 2002;126:1277–80.
62. Press RD, Bauer KA, Kujovich JL, et al. Clinical utility of factor V leiden (R506Q) testing for the diagnosis and management of thromboembolic disorders. Arch Pathol Lab Med 2002;126:1304–18.
63. McGlennen RC, Key NS. Clinical and laboratory management of the prothrombin G20210A mutation. Arch Pathol Lab Med 2002;126:1319–25.
64. Kottke-Marchant K, Comp P. Laboratory issues in diagnosing abnormalities of protein C, thrombomodulin, and endothelial cell protein C receptor. Arch Pathol Lab Med 2002;126:1337–48.
65. Goodwin AJ, Rosendaal FR, Kottke-Marchant K, et al. A review of the technical, diagnostic, and epidemiologic considerations for protein S assays. Arch Pathol Lab Med 2002;126:1349–66.
66. Kottke-Marchant K, Duncan A. Antithrombin deficiency: issues in laboratory diagnosis. Arch Pathol Lab Med 2002;126:1326–36.
67. Ridker PM, Miletich JP, Hennekens CH, et al. Ethnic distribution of factor V Leiden in 4047 men and women. Implications for venous thromboembolism screening. JAMA 1997;277:1305–7.
68. Chang MH, Lindegren ML, Butler MA, et al. Prevalence in the United States of selected candidate gene variants: Third National Health and Nutrition Examination Survey, 1991–1994. Am J Epidemiol 2009;169:54–66.
69. Dowling NF, Austin H, Dilley A, et al. The epidemiology of venous thromboembolism in Caucasians and African-Americans: the GATE Study. J Thromb Haemost 2003;1:80–7.

70. Patnaik MM, Moll S. Inherited antithrombin deficiency: a review. Haemophilia 2008;14:1229–39.
71. Miletich J, Sherman L, Broze G Jr. Absence of thrombosis in subjects with heterozygous protein C deficiency. N Engl J Med 1987;317:991–6.
72. Beauchamp NJ, Dykes AC, Parikh N, et al. The prevalence of, and molecular defects underlying, inherited protein S deficiency in the general population. Br J Haematol 2004;125:647–54.
73. Kupferminc MJ, Fait G, Many A, et al. Severe preeclampsia and high frequency of genetic thrombophilic mutations. Obstet Gynecol 2000;96:45–9.
74. Nagy B, Toth T, Rigo J Jr, et al. Detection of factor V Leiden mutation in severe pre-eclamptic Hungarian women. Clin Genet 1998;53:478–81.
75. Livingston JC, Barton JR, Park V, et al. Maternal and fetal inherited thrombophilias are not related to the development of severe preeclampsia. Am J Obstet Gynecol 2001;185:153–7.
76. Kupferminc MJ, Peri H, Zwang E, et al. High prevalence of the prothrombin gene mutation in women with intrauterine growth retardation, abruptio placentae and second trimester loss. Acta Obstet Gynecol Scand 2000;79:963–7.
77. Martinelli I, Taioli E, Cetin I, et al. Mutations in coagulation factors in women with unexplained late fetal loss. N Engl J Med 2000;343:1015–8.
78. Grandone E, Margaglione M, Colaizzo D, et al. Factor V Leiden is associated with repeated and recurrent unexplained fetal losses. Thromb Haemost 1997;77:822–4.

Hereditary Breast and Ovarian Cancer (HBOC): Clinical Features and Counseling for BRCA1 and BRCA2, Lynch Syndrome, Cowden Syndrome, and Li-Fraumeni Syndrome

Lee P. Shulman, MD[a,b,c,d,e,f],*

KEYWORDS

- Hereditary breast cancer • Hereditary ovarian cancer
- *BRCA1/2* • Genetic counseling • Lynch syndrome

Recent committee opinions from the Society of Gynecologic Oncologists[1] and The American College of Obstetricians and Gynecologists[2] highlight the need for cancer risk assessment to be a process in which genetic counseling plays a seminal role. It is the role of the genetic counselor to obtain relevant information concerning an individual's risk, to explain the process to the patient, explain how family history and laboratory testing provide an adjusted risk for developing cancer, and finally, to provide a lucid

This work is supported in part by the generosity of the Bears' Care Foundation.

[a] Division of Clinical Genetics, Feinberg School of Medicine of Northwestern University, Chicago, IL, USA

[b] Northwestern Ovarian Cancer Early Detection and Prevention Program, Feinberg School of Medicine of Northwestern University, Chicago, IL, USA

[c] Department of Obstetrics and Gynecology, Feinberg School of Medicine of Northwestern University, Chicago, IL, USA

[d] Cancer Genetics Program, Feinberg School of Medicine of Northwestern University, Chicago, IL, USA

[e] Robert H. Lurie Comprehensive Cancer Program, Feinberg School of Medicine of Northwestern University, Chicago, IL, USA

[f] University of Illinois at Chicago College of Pharmacy, Chicago, IL, USA

* Prentice Women's Hospital, 250 East, Superior Street, Room 05-2174, Chicago, IL 60611.

E-mail address: lps5@cornell.edu

Obstet Gynecol Clin N Am 37 (2010) 109–133
doi:10.1016/j.ogc.2010.03.003
0889-8545/10/$ – see front matter © 2010 Elsevier Inc. All rights reserved.

explanation of the risk for cancer development along with the preventative, screening, and diagnostic processes that are available to the patient based on the adjusted risk. It is indeed a complex and challenging task, given the emotional and psychosocial factors that affect the entire process and that must be addressed by the counselor.

The development and implementation of genetic counseling has been, until recently, mostly geared to pediatric, infertility, and prenatal issues. Counseling was initially based on mathematical algorithms (Bayesian analysis) that calculated the likelihood that a child or fetus would be affected; no specific prenatal testing was available and in many situations, the eventual pediatric diagnosis was based on phenotypic presentation or crude analyte measurement rather than a molecular assay. As such, disparate conditions with similar phenotypic presentations were classified as being manifestations of a similar disorder, eventually leading to inaccurate evaluations and counseling. While an important element of counseling was and remains emotional support for the patient, in many cases this was all that could be offered to those who had had an adverse perinatal or pediatric outcome, and were seeking reassurance and accurate evaluations for future children and other family members.

As understanding of the pathophysiology of diseases and disorders improved, genetic counseling began to provide more detailed and accurate assessment of the risk for particular conditions in future pregnancies and children. However, it was the development of ultrasound and amniocentesis that allowed for prenatal diagnosis, and thus more accurate counseling, to be provided to prospective parents. This further expanded with the delineation of the molecular basis for certain genetic disorders such as sickle cell disease and cystic fibrosis. Indeed, it was this step that laid the foundation for moving genetic counseling away from mathematical estimations of pediatric and prenatal risk to a more accurate assessment of risk for an increasing number of prenatal, pediatric, and adult conditions, thus changing the overall approach and use of genetic counseling in the evolving evidence-based approach to health care.

We now arrive at the current role of genetic counseling, and in particular, cancer genetic counseling. The completion of the Human Genome Project provided a virtual dictionary of gene and DNA sequences, all serving as a template for determining which sequences were associated with a variety of diseases as well as particular traits and characteristics. One disease state that was likely to be highly amenable to not only this new information but to the evolving and emerging technologies used to gather and interpret this molecular information was cancer. This article provides an overview of the molecular changes associated with inherited gynecologic malignancies and the incorporation of this information in the counseling of individuals at increased risk for developing malignancies, as well as conventional and emerging approaches to the screening of the general population.

The author examines cancer genetic counseling and its role in women's health care. The focus is hereditary breast and ovarian cancer (HBOC); however, cancer predisposition caused by genes other than *BRCA1/2* is also considered. The aim is to provide the reader with a foundation for counseling based on fundamental knowledge of the genes and their clinical consequences. The reader is then guided through the mechanics of risk assessment for individual patients, concluding with the psychosocial implications of counseling.

THE GENES AND BIOLOGY
Tumor Suppressor Genes

Two separate and distinct tumor suppressor genes, *BRCA1* and *BRCA2*, account for the approximately 85% of all cases of hereditary breast and epithelial ovarian cancer

(EOC),[3] although these 2 genes account for a smaller percentage of isolated familial breast cancer cases in the absence of EOC.[4] BRCA1 is located on chromosome 17q21, contains 22 coding exons, and spans 80 kb DNA, and BRCA2 is located on chromosome 13q12-13, contains 26 coding exons, and spans 70 kb DNA. Both genes are part of the DNA break repair pathway and appear to function as tumor suppressor genes, with mutations resulting in a highly penetrant susceptibility to the development of breast cancer and EOC. Mutations of BRCA1 and BRCA2 associated with the development of both malignancies are found throughout the coding regions and at splice sites, with most of these mutations being small insertions or deletions that lead to frameshift mutations, nonsense mutations, or splice site alterations. All of these genetic alterations invariably lead to premature protein termination and altered or absent proteins that fail to suppress the development of malignancies in breast and ovarian/epithelial tissues. In addition to these mutations and some missense mutations, large deletions and rearrangements not detectable by standard polymerase chain reaction (PCR) have recently been identified and are now part of the molecular testing provided to those undergoing genetic testing for BRCA mutations. Palma and colleagues[5] reported that genomic rearrangements, detected by an analysis separate from conventional gene sequencing and aimed at detecting large gene rearrangements not amenable to detection by conventional analyses[6] (eg, BART analysis [BRACAnalysis Rearrangement Test]), accounted for 18% of BRCA1/2 mutations in non-Ashkenazi Jewish probands with no such rearrangements being detected in Ashkenazi Jewish probands.

The frequency of BRCA1 or BRCA2 mutations in the general population is estimated to be 1 in 300 to 1 in 800,[7] though a more recent study by Risch and colleagues[8] in Canada suggest that these frequencies may be considerably higher, at 1 in 140 to 1 in 300. However, some populations and communities have a higher frequency of certain BRCA1/2 mutations than is found in the general population. In the United States, BRCA1/2 mutations are found in approximately 1 of every 40 individuals of Eastern European (Ashkenazi) Jewish ancestry. What also distinguishes this community is that 3 mutations (185delAG and 5382insC in BRCA1 and 6174delT in BRCA2) account for approximately 98% of mutations detected.[9] In Iceland, the 999del5 mutation in BRCA2 accounts for approximately 7% of all cases of EOC occurring in Icelanders.[10] These mutations are known as "founder mutations," so named because in certain populations begun by a small ancestral group isolated by societal behavior or geography, certain genes in the original "founders" of a community or population can become far more common in succeeding generations after initiation of the isolation than would occur in the general population. The identification of founder mutations allows for more facile screening of individuals of those groups associated with these mutations. As such, evaluating individuals of Eastern European Jewish ancestry at increased risk for a BRCA1 or BRCA2 mutation based on family history is now accomplished by first determining the presence of one of these 3 mutations unless analysis of an affected relative shows that the BRCA1/2 mutation in the family is not one of these 3 mutations. Evaluating for these 3 mutations in high-risk members of the Ashkenazi Jewish community is not only easier than gene sequencing but also less costly. However, even in some clinical scenarios in which a single putative BRCA1/2 mutation is of interest in the risk assessment process, a "single site" analysis would potentially be augmented with a founder mutation analysis or even full gene sequencing if the family history indicates that another mutation may be present, possibly from the other parental lineage. For individuals from populations associated with founder mutations who are at increased risk for BRCA1/2 mutations based on family history and found not to have one of the founder mutations, gene sequencing and rearrangement analysis can be offered after a "negative" result to provide a complete and thorough molecular evaluation.

Mismatch Repair Genes

Lynch syndrome (LS) is caused by gene mutations in the multistep mismatch repair (MMR) system. MMR genes are located on 5 different chromosomes and encode for proteins that recognize and repair damage in the DNA that leads to DNA mismatches. One complex of proteins consisting of the protein MSH2 combined with MSH6 or MSH3 recognizes the DNA mismatch and binds to the site. An inactivating mutation of MSH2 blocks the ability to recognize a DNA mismatch, negating the function of this complex. Mutations of either MSH6 or MSH3, on the other hand, may not have a similar deleterious effect as these 2 proteins have overlapping functions, and thus an inactivating or adverse mutation in one may not adversely affect the function of the overall MMR system. Once a mismatch is recognized, MLH1 (with PMS1 or PMS2) then provides the necessary steps to resynthesize the DNA strand in its original and correct sequence.

A total of 7 MMR enzymes have been delineated, and mutations in each of the 7 genes have been identified (**Table 1**).[11] Mutations in the MLH1 and MSH2 genes make up approximately 90% of observed mutations in MMR genes and are followed next by mutations in MSH6 and PMS2. Mutations in the remaining 3 genes are not commonly observed in LS families. The type of MMR mutation provides important information as to the risk for developing a particular malignancy in women with LS mutations. While MLH1 and MSH2 gene mutations are the most common mutations found in cases of colorectal cancer (CRC), Wijnen and colleagues[12] found that women carrying MSH6 mutations were twice as likely to develop endometrial cancer as women who carried MSH2 or MLH1 mutations, and Watson and colleagues[13] reported that the risk for EOC was significantly higher in families with MSH2 mutations compared with families with MLH1 mutations.

It is interesting that the mechanism by which MMR gene mutations predispose to tumor development appear to differ from the loss of heterozygosity observed in HBOC. Aaltonen and colleagues[14] found no loss of heterozygosity at a locus coinciding with the MSH2 site on chromosome 2 linked to colorectal cancer in 14 cases from 3 families, strongly suggestive of a molecular mechanism for LS different from biallelic inactivation and alteration of tumor-suppressing gene function in cancer susceptibility syndromes such as HBOC. Another explanation may be that MMR mutations adversely affect the DNA mismatch repair mechanism without the loss of heterozygosity, thus leading to a "domino-like" cascade on those cellular

Table 1
MMR genes associated with mismatch repair system

Gene Name	Mutation Frequency in LS pts	Chromosome Locus
MLH1	40%–45%	3p21.3
MSH2	40%–45%	2p22-p21
MSH6	7%–10%	2p16
PMS1	Unknown	2q31-q33
PMS2	<5%	7p22
MSH3	0	5q11-q12
MLH3	0	14q24.3

mechanisms responsible for the maintenance of proper cellular growth and development, and thus predisposing those targeted cells and organs to malignant transformation with a mechanism different than that observed in HBOC. These inactivating mutations not only prevent the repair of damaged DNA but also increase the rate of mutations at the DNA microsatellites of growth-regulating genes. Microsatellites are short (1–5 base pairs), polymorphic DNA sequences that are repeated 15 to 30 times at a given locus and are distributed throughout the genome. Microsatellite instability (MSI) thus serves as a marker for MMR mutations; indeed, microsatellite instability analysis and immunohistochemical (IHC) staining for the presence or absence of the proteins MLH1, MSH2, MSH6, and PMS2 serve as preliminary diagnostic steps in determining the presence of a DNA repair defect for many individuals at increased risk for MMR mutations. IHC can evaluate tumor tissue for gene expression but cannot assess the functionality of any of these proteins. As such, IHC alone cannot determine whether the protein present does not function properly because of a missense mutation; accordingly, IHC should be combined with MSI to screen prospective tumors for MMR mutations. MSI is a common feature of LS-associated tumors; however, studies of MSI in ovarian tumor tissue from EOC have not provided consistent diagnostic correlation.

CLINICAL FEATURES
Hereditary Breast and Ovarian Cancer

HBOC syndrome is one of the most common reasons for referral for genetic counseling and consideration of genetic testing. HBOC is characterized by a strong family history of breast cancer and EOC, with most such families having more cases of breast cancer than ovarian cancer. HBOC families, like other families with hereditary cancer predisposition syndromes, are characterized by a far earlier age of onset than is seen in the general population, as well as a higher likelihood of bilateral disease. In addition, HBOC families have a markedly higher frequency of family members with breast cancer and EOC occurring in the same individual and, for some gene mutations, a strikingly higher risk for breast cancer in men.

A study by Ramus and Gayther[15] showed that 81% of families with at least 2 cases of EOC and 1 case of breast cancer had a deleterious mutation in BRCA1 or BRCA2, thus confirming earlier studies and models demonstrating that the majority of cases of HBOC are associated with BRCA1/2 mutations.[16,17] Indeed, Lynch and colleagues[3] reported that BRCA1/2 mutations were found in approximately 6% to 8% of isolated EOC cases, but in 80% to 90% of HBOC cases.

As BRCA1 and BRCA2 are autosomal genes with high penetrance, transmission can occur either maternally or paternally; accordingly, equal attention must be paid to the assessment of paternal relatives of an individual being evaluated for a possible BRCA1/2 mutation. BRCA1 mutations have not been shown to consistently increase risk for breast cancer in men whereas BRCA2 mutations have been shown to increase the risk for male breast cancer. Accordingly, any case of male breast cancer, regardless of age at diagnosis, should prompt the offering of genetic counseling and consideration of genetic testing for HBOC because of the overall low frequency of male breast cancer in the general population and the markedly increased risk in men with BRCA2 mutations. Kessler and colleagues (personal communication, 2007) found that among individuals at increased risk for heritable colon cancer, an equal distribution of paternal and maternal transmission of deleterious (and autosomal) genes was found. However, among individuals at increased risk for HBOC, an approximately 70:30 (maternal to paternal) distribution was found when an equal ratio would have been predicted (*BRCA1/2* are autosomal). Families with either few members or few females pose a barrier to accurate risk assessment, as affected females provide the main evidence of the existence of a deleterious *BRCA1/2* mutation. Kessler's study (personal communication) shows that in many cases, affected females in the paternal lineage are either ignored or not considered on an equal basis with affected members from the maternal lineage because of a misperception that HBOC is a disease of women, and that genetic events in the paternal families of putative *BRCA1/2* mutation carriers do not play as important a role in the assessment of risk as those affected individuals in the maternal lineage.

Mutations in *BRCA1/2* confer a markedly increased risk for developing breast cancer and EOC, with *BRCA1* and *BRCA2* mutations both being associated with an approximately 85% to 90% risk for developing breast cancer by the age of 70 (**Figs. 1** and **2**).[18,19] However, whereas *BRCA1/2* mutations are associated with a markedly elevated risk for developing EOC, *BRCA1* mutations are associated with a higher risk for developing EOC than *BRCA2* mutations (see **Figs. 1** and **2**). Risch and colleagues[20] found 60 germline mutations in *BRCA1/2* among 649 unselected cases of EOC; 39 were in *BRCA1* and 21 in *BRCA2*. Satagopan and colleagues[21] found that carriers of either of the 2 *BRCA1* founder mutations in the Ashkenazi Jewish population (185delAG and 5382insC) were estimated to have a 37% risk for developing EOC by the age of 70 years, whereas those carrying the founder *BRCA2* mutation (6174delT) were estimated to have a 21% risk. Other clinical differences between the 2 *BRCA1/2* gene mutations include an approximately 100-fold increased risk for male breast cancer among *BRCA2* mutation carriers with only a potentially slight increased risk for male breast cancer among *BRCA1* mutation carriers.[22] In addition, an increased risk for early-onset prostate and pancreatic cancer among *BRCA2* mutation carriers has been observed in some studies,[8,23] whereas other studies of high-risk prostate cancer families have observed little impact of *BRCA2* mutations.[24] In addition, a marked increased risk for pancreatic and gastric cancers in *BRCA1* mutation carriers has been reported[25]; of interest is that Risch and colleagues[8] similarly reported an increased risk for pancreatic and gastric cancers in *BRCA1* and *BRCA2* carriers, although they found the risk for pancreatic cancer to be higher among *BRCA2* carriers and the risk for gastric cancer to be higher in *BRCA1* carriers. Finally, although most of the morbidity and mortality associated with *BRCA1/2* mutations has

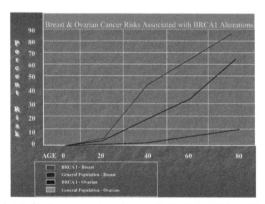

Fig. 1. Age-related risk for breast and ovarian cancers associated with *BRCA1* mutations. (*Adapted from* Brose MS, Rebbeck TR, Calzone KA, et al. Cancer risk estimates for *BRCA1* mutation carriers. J Natl Cancer Inst 2002;94:1365–72; with permission.)

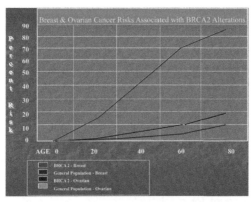

Fig. 2. Age-related risk for breast and ovarian cancers associated with *BRCA2* mutations. (*Adapted from* The Breast Cancer Linkage Consortium. Cancer risks in *BRCA2* mutation carriers. J Natl Cancer Inst 1999;91(15):1310–6; with permission.)

been focused on the increased risk for breast and ovarian cancers and other malignancies, Mai and colleagues[26] report a significantly increased risk for noncancer mortality among *BRCA1/2* mutation carriers, thus potentially adding another considerable medical and emotional issue to be addressed by genetic counselors providing counseling to individuals at increased risk for having *BRCA1/2* mutations.

Lynch Syndrome

CRC is the third most common type of cancer in the United States, with more than 140,000 new cases diagnosed each year. LS is the most common hereditary form of CRC and is believed to account for up to 3% of all cases; with this projected frequency of 1 out of every 35 individuals with CRC having LS, more than 28,000 new cases of LS will occur worldwide in 2010.[27] This does not include individuals at increased risk for CRC because of a positive family history; familial CRC, defined as 2 or more first-degree relatives with CRC, is thought to account for up to 20% of all cases of CRC.[27] If the impact of germline mutations and family history affect the frequency of CRC and associated malignancies to this degree, the failure to assess family history and to identify at-risk individuals to allow for earlier detection and intervention programs clearly places a considerable number of people at risk for developing malignancies that could have ostensibly been prevented. As such, the value of genetic counseling and testing for LS in at-risk individuals seems to be a relatively straightforward and important step in reducing the risk for CRC and other associated Lynch malignancies.

As with other cancer susceptibility syndromes, LS is associated with an increased risk for cancers in multiple organs including endometrial, urogenital, pancreatic and biliary tract, and EOC. Of note is that more recent study of Lynch families shows that female members of these families have a higher cumulative lifetime risk for developing endometrial cancer than for developing colorectal cancer.[27] Women who carry a germline mutation for LS have a 20% to 60% lifetime risk of developing endometrial cancer; Aarnio and colleagues[28] reported standardized incidence ratios of 68% and 62%, respectively, in LS individuals with mutations in *MLH1* or *MSH2*. Banno and colleagues[29] reported the frequency of microsatellite instability markers among 38 cases of endometrial cancers from individuals with familial clustering of cancers (endometrial and other cancers) to be 31.6%, and Mathews and colleagues[30] found immunohistochemical evidence of mismatch repair deficiency in 34% of newly diagnosed endometrial cancer patients younger than 50 years, indicating an important pathophysiological role for abnormal DNA mismatch repair in the pathogenesis of endometrial cancer. Counselors and clinicians who care for women with endometrial cancer or their families must thus be mindful of the potential for LS in women with endometrial cancer, especially those with family histories of other LS-associated malignancies or with clinical presentations that would be suggestive of a heritable predisposition to cancer development (eg, early age of diagnosis).

Watson and colleagues[13] reported the lifetime risk (up to age 70 years) for extracolonic tumors among a total of over 6000 LS mutation carriers, probable mutation carriers (with CRC and/or endometrial cancer), and first-degree relatives of these 2 cohorts to be 8.4% for urologic tract cancers, with risks higher for males and *MSH2* families. Despite the high risk for developing EOC among women with or at risk for LS, LS mutations account for a relatively small proportion of all cases of EOC.[31] EOCs associated with *BRCA1/2* mutations are mostly serous in nature; however, LS mutations are associated with a variety of ovarian cancer epithelial malignancies including endometrioid and clear cell cancers. Of note, while most cases of ovarian cancer in LS families are malignant epithelial tumors, most are well or moderately differentiated and are International Federation of Gynecology and Obstetrics (FIGO) Stage I or II at the time of diagnosis. This is in sharp contrast to *BRCA* mutation-associated tumors, which tend to present in a more advanced stage and be more poorly differentiated. Most of the Lynch families with EOC who were studied were found to have germline mutations of the MLH1 or MSH2 genes.[32] However, Cederquist and colleagues[33] reported a high frequency of a variety of EOC in Swedish women with MSH6 mutations, with an estimated 33% lifetime risk of developing EOC in this Swedish cohort. As with other cancer susceptibility genes, certain mutations in particular populations may exert a different impact on cancer risk than that typically observed in the general population (ie, founder mutations). However, similar to women with *BRCA1/2* mutations, women with Lynch mutations tend to develop EOC at a younger age (fifth decade) than sporadic cases of EOC (seventh decade). Watson and colleagues[13] also reported cases of cancers of the brain, small bowel, stomach, biliary tract, and breast in their cohort, though with considerably lower frequencies.

The diagnosis of LS is made by detecting a mutation in an *MMR* gene.[27] While there is little controversy concerning increased surveillance for carriers of MMR mutations, there is controversy concerning the approach to screening for such mutations. This controversy revolves around uncertainties regarding whether the prevalence of *MMR* mutations is sufficient to warrant large-scale screening, the trade-offs between screening all patients with CRC versus targeted screening of certain high-risk groups characterized by early age of diagnosis, family history, and tumor histology, and whether to recommend immunohistochemistry (IHC) or MSI as the primary screening tool.[34] As such, unlike the detection of *BRCA1/2* mutations, it is not the standard of care to test every CRC or Lynch-associated cancer patient for germline mutations in the *MMR* genes. It is currently recommended that a comprehensive family history of cancers of all anatomic sites be obtained, with attention paid to the cardinal features of LS.

ASSESSING CANCER RISK

Cancer risk assessment is a process by which individuals are identified who are at increased risk for a hereditary or familial cancer and are offered a different approach to prevention and screening than that which is offered to individuals in the general population. Such altered interventions for high-risk individuals can range from an earlier initiation of screening, such as the initiation of mammography before the age of 40 years in women with a *BRCA1/2* mutation, to the incorporation of screening protocols not offered to non–high-risk individuals, such as the use of regular breast magnetic resonance imaging (MRI) examinations in women with *BRCA1/2* mutations. The detection of a deleterious mutation may also prompt a novel or unique approach to prevention, such as the consideration of oral contraceptive use to reduce the risk for EOC in women with *BRCA1/2* mutations, prophylactic colectomy in individuals with mutations in DNA repair genes (LS), and prophylactic premenopausal salpingoophor-ectomy in women with *BRCA1/2* mutations. However, not all preventative measures offered to high-risk individuals are necessarily extreme or extirpative in nature; for example, women at increased risk for EOC are likely to be encouraged to breastfeed or consider bilateral tubal ligation once childbearing has been completed as a way to reduce the risk for EOC without increasing the risk for breast cancer.[4,35] What is clear is that the identification of high-risk individuals, whether as result of inheriting a delete-rious mutation or because of a extensive family history of cancer, allows for the offering of risk reduction strategies that have been shown to prolong lives and improve quality of life for high-risk individuals.[36] This is the rationale for the current approach to cancer genetic counseling and risk assessment.

HBOC

Until an inexpensive and facile method becomes available that provides information on an individual's complete genome, there will controversies as to who is offered genetic counseling and genetic testing to determine whether a deleterious mutation in a tumor suppressor gene in present and is adversely affecting risk of developing malignancy. The United States Preventative Services Task Force (USPSTF) put forth guidelines in 2005[37] recommending that only women at high risk for having a delete-rious *BRCA1/2* mutation be offered counseling and testing. The USPSTF defined high-risk women as those non-Ashkenazi Jewish women with 2 first-degree relatives with breast cancer, 1 of whom received the diagnosis at age 50 years or younger; a combi-nation of 3 or more first- or second-degree relatives with breast cancer regardless of age at diagnosis; a combination of both breast and ovarian cancer among first- and second-degree relatives; a first-degree relative with bilateral breast cancer; a combi-nation of 2 or more first- or second-degree relatives with ovarian cancer regardless of age at diagnosis; a first- or second-degree relative with both breast and ovarian cancer at any age; and a history of breast cancer in a male relative. For women of Ashkenazi Jewish heritage, an increased-risk family history includes any first-degree relative (or 2 second-degree relatives on the same side of the family) with breast or ovarian cancer. Based on these criteria, it was estimated that about 2% of adult women in the general population have an increased-risk family history and should be offered counseling and testing. Women with none of these family history patterns have a low probability of having a deleterious mutation in *BRCA1* or *BRCA2* genes, and the routine offer of counseling and testing to such low-risk individuals is not recommended.

The USPSTF guidelines are just one attempt to quantify risk and identify those indi-viduals who would most benefit from counseling and genetic testing. Other approaches to quantifying risk include the popular Gail Model, as well as *BRCA* Pro and the most recent breast cancer risk assessment tool from the National Cancer Institute, the Breast Cancer Assessment Tool (www.cancer.gov; **Table 2**). All of these methods are meant to be used by clinicians to determine breast cancer risk and take

Table 2
Questions in the Breast Cancer Assessment Tool from the National Cancer Institute, last modified April 28, 2008 (Click a question number for a brief explanation, or read all explanations)

1. Does the woman have a medical history of any breast cancer or of ductal carcinoma in situ (DCIS) or lobular carcinoma in situ (LCIS)?	Select ▼
2. What is the woman's age? *This tool only calculates risk for women 35 years of age or older*	Select ▼
3. What was the woman's age at the time of her first menstrual period?	Select ▼
4. What was the woman's age at the time of her first live birth of a child?	Select ▼
5. How many of the woman's first-degree relatives—mother, sisters, daughters—have had breast cancer?	Select ▼
6. Has the woman ever had a breast biopsy?	Select ▼
6a. How many breast biopsies (positive or negative) has the woman had?	Select ▼
6b. Has the woman had at least one breast biopsy with atypical hyperplasia?	Select ▼
7. What is the woman's race/ethnicity?	Select ▼

From Available at: http://www.cancer.gov. Accessed March 1, 2010.

into account a variety of demographic, family and personal history, and medical history to arrive at an adjusted risk for developing breast cancer. Indeed, newer risk assessment tools include factors other than personal and family history and are considered to provide a more accurate assessment of risk by including such parameters as breast density, measurements of serum estradiol and androgens, body mass index, and history of fracture and height loss.[38] Those women found to be at increased risk, usually considered to be a lifetime breast cancer risk of 20% to 25% or greater, are typically offered counseling and genetic testing, as well as different screening interventions such as annual breast MRI examinations.

Recent guidelines from the American College of Obstetricians and Gynecologists[2] and the Society of Gynecologic Oncologists[1] have clarified the need for clinicians to incorporate risk assessment into their practices to identify those women who may benefit from counseling and testing. Although these guidelines and recommendations do not promote a more expansive role for genetic testing, they do raise awareness of the marked increased risk of cancer development in individuals with tumor suppressor gene mutations and with family members with certain malignancies. The guidelines thus serve to encourage clinicians to incorporate cancer risk assessment, ranging from a detailed family history to the use of a risk assessment tool such as the Gail model or the Breast Cancer Risk Assessment Tool, and provide individuals at increased risk for cancer to consider counseling, testing, and more appropriate screening options. In this regard it is hoped that if such recommendations increase the number of people undergoing genetic testing, it is as result of more people at high risk recognizing their increased risk for developing cancer, and clinicians choosing to further evaluate this risk with genetic testing rather than a greater (and inappropriate) concern for developing such malignancies in the low-risk population.

Lynch Syndrome

Assessing an individual or a family for LS is accomplished by determining whether the history meets Amsterdam II criteria (**Table 3**). If a family history is suggestive of LS but the criteria cannot be met because of family size or other factors, consideration of risk can be accomplished using revised Bethesda criteria (**Table 4**). Women with Lynch mutations do not have a marked increased risk for developing breast cancer; as such, family histories with multiple family members with ovarian cancer and no cases of breast cancer, but having family members with Lynch-associated malignancies (eg, colorectal cancer, endometrial cancer) should first be evaluated for *MMR* mutations rather than *BRCA1/2* mutations.[39]

Individuals who meet Amsterdam II criteria are evaluated by obtaining peripheral blood for direct sequencing of the MLH1 and MSH2 genes. For those individuals whose families do not meet Amsterdam criteria but do meet Bethesda criteria, first evaluating tumor tissue for MSI and IHC (before mutation testing) is the preferred approach for screening at-risk individuals. MSI testing and IHC appear to provide concordant information, as Vasen and colleagues[40] reported a 93% concordance between the 2 tests in colon cancer specimens. This approach is associated with high (90%–95%) sensitivity for detecting *MMR* gene mutation carriers,[34] but as with IHC, it provides no information as to which gene is mutated and thus which malignancy that individual may have the highest risk for developing. As such, the diagnosis of LS currently proceeds in a stepwise approach[27]:

1. Clinical suspicion from early-onset cancer or family history
2. Amsterdam II criteria assessment. If positive, germline mutation testing. If negative,
3. Bethesda criteria. If positive,
4. MSI testing. If MSI-High (MSI-H), germline mutation testing.

Unfortunately, Amsterdam II and Bethesda criteria have limitations for identifying individuals at increased risk for LS. Both sets of criteria are based on CRC being the preeminent malignancy; while the new criteria do recognize the role of extracolonic malignancies, it is not clear how these criteria would work in the context of an individual or family presenting with extracolonic malignancies but not CRC. While Bethesda criteria work best to determine which tumors require further testing, individuals with small pedigrees as well as those with a predominance of familial endometrial cancer may not be well served by even these more recent guidelines.[41]

Table 3 Amsterdam II criteria for Lynch syndrome	
At least 3 relatives with an HNPCC cancer:	Colorectal, endometrial, stomach, ovary, ureter/renal pelvis, brain, small intestine, hepatobiliary tract, or sebaceous tumor of skin
AND: • One is a first-degree relative of the other 2 • At least 2 successive generations affected • At least 1 of the HNPCC cancers was diagnosed at <50 y • Familial adenomatous polyposis has been excluded	

Abbreviation: HNPCC, hereditary nonpolyposis colorectal cancer.

Table 4
Bethesda guidelines to determine which colorectal tumors should undergo MSI testing
Colorectal cancer diagnosed in a patient <50 y, or
Presence of synchronous or metachronous colorectal, or other HNPCC-associated tumor, regardless of age, or
Colorectal cancer with the MSI-H histology diagnosed in patient <60 y, or
Colorectal cancer or HNPCC-tumor diagnosed <50 y in at least 1 first-degree relative, or
Colorectal cancer or HNPCC-associated tumor diagnosed at any age in 2 first-degree or second-degree relatives

Another approach to screening individuals for LS is presented by the Society of Gynecologic Oncologists (SGO), which combines some of the aforementioned issues into the following committee report[1] (adapted from Table 1 of Resnick and colleagues[41]).

For patients with a 20% to 25% risk of LS, genetic risk assessment is strongly recommended. Such patients include:

- Family pedigrees meeting Amsterdam criteria
- Patients with metachronous (define) or synchronous (define) CRC, endometrial cancer or ovarian cancer before age 50
- Individuals with a first- or second-degree relative with a known germline mutation in a mismatch repair gene.

For patients with a 5% to 10% risk for LS, genetic risk assessment may be helpful. Such patients include:

- Patients with CRC or endometrial cancer diagnosed before age 50
- Patients with endometrial and/or ovarian cancer and a synchronous or metachronous Lynch-associated tumor at any age
- Patients with CRC or endometrial cancer and a first-degree relative diagnosed with a Lynch-associated malignancy before age 50
- Patients with CRC or endometrial cancer at any age with 2 or more first- or second-degree relatives diagnosed with a Lynch-associated malignancy at any age
- A patient with a first- or second-degree relative who meets the above criteria.

While the SGO recommendations present a clear identification of who may benefit from genetic risk assessment and testing, they does not provide insight into what testing should be offered.[41] At present, colon cancer MSI testing and IHC are used to triage patients to determine who should receive counseling and consideration of gene sequencing, with IHC being an efficient and cost-effective tool in identifying tumors with mismatch repair deficiency. However, the lack of emphasis on gynecologic malignancies in the Amsterdam II and Bethesda criteria, as well as the recognition that having an age cut-off of 50 years below which IHC testing is routinely applied to endometrial cancer cases, may be too low to adequately identify a sufficient number of individuals with LS who present with endometrial cancer[42,43] leads one to consider an alternative approach to risk assessment and genetic testing for putative LS individuals with endometrial cancer. Resnick and colleagues[41] propose a screening algorithm with endometrial cancer cases that uses an age cut-off of 60 years rather than 50 years to determine which specimens are to be tested by IHC for MLH1,

MSH2, MSH6, and PMS2. Of the 1 in 5 specimens that have an abnormal IHC from this expanded initial cohort, and adding to this individuals with considerable family histories or evidence of Cowden syndrome (see later discussion), approximately 12% of cases would be referred for genetic counseling and gene sequencing.

Although there is currently no standard or conventional approach to either the identification of individuals at increased risk or screening and testing of those individuals who may have inherited a mutated *MMR* gene, future technological advances, including microarray assays, may make the development of diagnostic criteria or screening algorithms obsolete. One of the major drawbacks to large-scale mutation screening is the time and cost of such testing. The development of accurate and less costly molecular analyses will surely promote a more widespread use of gene testing for at-risk individuals for LS and other cancer susceptibility conditions.

OTHER HEREDITARY CANCER SYNDROMES INVOLVING BREAST AND GYNECOLOGIC MALIGNANCIES
Cowden Syndrome

Cowden syndrome, or multiple hamartoma syndrome, is an autosomal dominant condition characterized by the formation of multiple hamartomas in any organ of the body and an increased risk for cancer. Pathognomonic features of Cowden syndrome include facial trichilemmomas, acral keratosis, and oral papillomatous papules Individuals with Cowden syndrome are at increased risk for developing a variety of benign and malignant conditions, with more than 90% of individuals demonstrating mucocutaneous lesions.[44] Germline mutations in PTEN (*P*hosphatase and *TEN*sin homologue deleted on chromosome *TEN*), located at 10q23.3, have been found in 85% of Cowden syndrome individuals as well as in other rare and unrelated conditions such as Bannayan-Riley-Ruvalcaba syndrome and Proteus syndrome. However, these syndromes do share some common phenotypic features that have led to the characterization of these conditions under the common classification of PHTS (PTEN hamartoma tumor syndrome).[45]

In addition to the hamartomatous and dermatologic conditions, Cowden syndrome is associated with an increased risk of a variety of malignancies. Lifetime risk for non-medullary thyroid cancer is approximately 10%, with benign thyroid conditions also increased in prevalence among affected individuals. Lhermitte-Duclos disease (dysplastic gangliocytoma of the cerebellum) and renal cell carcinoma have also been reported to be components of Cowden syndrome, although the exact frequency of these 2 conditions among individuals with Cowden syndrome has not been well defined. An increased risk of breast cancer has been reported among men with Cowden syndrome.

Women with Cowden syndrome have an approximate 75% risk for benign breast disease such as fibromas, fibroadenomas, and fibrocystic changes, as well as a 25% to 50% lifetime risk for breast cancer.[43] In addition, women with Cowden syndrome have a 5% to 10% lifetime risk of endometrial cancer and an increased risk of developing uterine fibroids.

Diagnosis of Cowden syndrome is achieved by demonstrating major and minor criteria as put forth in the International Cowden Syndrome Consortium Operational Criteria for the Diagnosis of Cowden Syndrome.[46] Approximately 80% of individuals who meet the diagnostic criteria are found to have mutations in *PTEN*. Because of the considerable and varied increased risk for cancer development in individuals with Cowden syndrome, extraordinary surveillance should be provided to detect malignancies at an earlier and more treatable stage. Such screening may include a baseline thyroid examination and ultrasound at 18 years old with an annual thyroid examination thereafter. A family history of renal cancer should prompt an annual urinalysis and urine cytology along with a renal ultrasound. Women with Cowden syndrome should begin annual clinical breast examinations at age 18 years with semi-annual examinations beginning at age 25. Mammography should be offered at approximately 25 to 30 years, or 10 years earlier than the youngest affected female in the family. In addition, women with Cowden syndrome should be offered an annual breast MRI on initiation of annual mammographic examinations. Men with Cowden syndrome should have annual clinical breast examinations starting at age 25 to 30 years, with further evaluation based on the finding of palpable lesions. Annual endometrial biopsies should be performed starting at age 35 to 40 years, or 10 years earlier than the youngest affected individual in the family. This can also be augmented by an annual endovaginal ultrasound examination in postmenopausal women.[44] Endometrial cancer is amenable to risk reduction, and approaches to prevention should also be discussed with affected individuals. Such measures can include oral contraceptives and intrauterine devices to reduce the incidence of endometrial cancer as well as hysterectomy.[47]

Li-Fraumeni Syndrome

Li-Fraumeni syndrome (LFS) is a rare cancer predisposition syndrome estimated to account for approximately 1% of hereditary breast cancer cases. Mutations in TP53, a tumor suppressor gene located on 17p13.1, are the primary cause of LFS, which is transmitted in an autosomal dominant fashion. In addition, families with classic LFS phenotypes have also been found to have mutations in the CHEK2 gene, found on 22q12.2. Unlike TP53, CHEK2 encodes for a serine/threonine protein kinase which phosphorylates p53, leading to cessation of mitosis and allowing DNA repair; CHEK2 mutations thus promote the development of malignancy by inhibiting DNA repair, similar to the MMR genes.

LFS is characterized by early-onset breast cancer, soft-tissue sarcomas, adrenocortical tumors, brain tumors, and leukemias. In some families with LFS, brain tumors, adrenocortical tumors, and sarcomas may present in childhood. Additional tumors reported in LFS families include ovary, pancreas, lung, stomach, melanoma, and Wilms tumor.[44] Similar to other cancer susceptibility conditions, LFS appears to increase the risk of early development of cancer, with a 50% risk of cancer by age 40 years and a 90% risk of cancer by age 60.[48] Screening and management of patients at risk for LFS is challenging given the variety of early-onset malignancies associated with this condition. In women, annual clinical breast examinations, including MRI and mammography, should start at age 20 years, and consideration of oral contraception use is warranted to reduce the risk of ovarian cancer, along with an annual pelvic and abdominal ultrasound examination. However, there are no published guidelines for screening LFS patients; clinicians should strongly consider genetic counseling and testing (TP53 and CHEK2) for individuals and family members with a considerable history of sarcomas and early-onset cancers.

Breast and other gynecologic cancers are found as associated malignancies in other genetic syndromes (**Table 5**), all of which are rare and associated with a varied spectrum of nonmalignant conditions and disorders. Syndromes associated with ovarian cancer are rare and are usually associated with nonepithelial ovarian cancer, although some cases of serous and mucinous EOC have been reported. Although ovarian cancers and tumors have been reported in women with these genetic conditions, the overall risk for developing EOC in women with these conditions seems to be similar to that of the general population. However, the risk for developing breast and

Table 5
Genetic syndromes associated with breast and gynecologic cancers

Syndrome	Inheritance	Gene (Chromosome)	Clinical Features	Gyn/Breast Cancer
Peutz-Jeghers	AD	STK11 (19)	Melanocytic macules (mouth and lips); polyps in GI tract; increased risk of GI tract carcinoma	Sex cord-stromal tumors; granulosa cell tumors; breast cancer
Ollier	Sporadic/AD?	PTHR1 (3)	Multiple enchondromas; secondary chondrosarcomas; orthopedic complications	Granulosa cell tumors
Gorlin	AD	PTCH (9)	Basal cell carcinoma of the skin before age 30; jaw cysts; vertebral abnormalities	Fibrosarcoma; also benign fibromas
Ataxia-telangiectasia	AR	ATM (11q22.3)	Delayed motor skill development, slurred speech, telangiectasias, ALL, lymphoma	Breast cancer in heterozygous state
Hereditary diffuse gastric cancer	AD	CDH1(16q22.1)	Early-onset gastric cancer	Lobular breast cancer
Li-Fraumeni	AD	TP53 (17p13) CHEK2 (22q12)	Early-onset multiple tumor types especially sarcomas, breast, brain adrenal, and leukemias	Breast cancer
Cowden	AD	PTEN (10q23)	Hamartomatous lesions especially skin, mucous membranes, breast, and thyroid	Breast cancer

Abbreviations: AD, autosomal dominant; ALL, acute lymphoblastic leukemia; AR, autosomal recessive; GI, gastrointestinal.

endometrial cancers may be increased in individuals affected with these syndromes. Notwithstanding, evaluation of the pelvis by ultrasound or laparoscopy in cases of pelvic masses, as well as mammography in affected women with breast masses, is warranted.

COUNSELING

The past 2 decades have witnessed the identification of several genes that have been associated with hereditable breast and gynecologic cancers, thereby promoting the development of and need for cancer genetic counseling. Similar to conventional genetic counseling for pediatric and prenatal conditions, cancer genetic counseling is geared to identifying individuals with cancer predisposition gene mutations as well as those family and personal histories that affect the overall risk for development of cancer. However, unlike conventional genetic counseling in which most individuals or fetuses with a particular phenotype are likely to possess a deleterious gene or abnormal chromosome complement, most cases of cancer, even those associated with considerable family histories in individuals of high-risk ethnic and racial groups, are not associated with the inheritance of cancer predisposition genes. Indeed, no more than 10% of most types of cancer are associated with heritable conditions.[49] Nonetheless, cancer genetic counseling has become a seminal part of the risk assessment process; not only to identify those individuals with mutations in cancer predisposition genes but also to reassure those individuals who have not inherited such mutations, as well as to counsel those individuals who have not inherited specific mutations but may still be at increased risk for developing malignancies.

The increased risk for developing cancer in women with mutations in cancer susceptibility genes invariably begins with the inheritance of a germline mutation within a tumor suppressor gene from either parent. Although gynecologic malignancies can only occur in females, genes that predispose to the development of gynecologic malignancies are usually autosomal in nature and thus can be inherited from either parent. This concept is critical with regard to family history information, as both parents can transmit deleterious gene mutations; accordingly, obtaining careful and detailed family histories of an individual's maternal and paternal families is vital to developing an accurate risk assessment for an individual.

By definition, a germline mutation is present at conception; every cell of the individual will have the gene mutation, a fact that is likely associated with the involvement of multiple organs in many cancer susceptibility syndromes. However, the inheritance of a mutated cancer susceptibility allele is only the *first* step (eg, 1 of 2 tumor suppressor genes with no mutations and 1 gene with a mutation) in promoting the development of a malignancy, and does not guarantee that an individual will go on to develop a particular malignancy. The development of a heritable cancer, as well as most other cancers, is postulated to be dependent on the occurrence of a second genomic alteration.[50] That an individual has inherited the first "step" serves to explain why such individuals have a considerably higher risk for developing cancer than the general population, as well as why cancer predisposition syndromes tend to present with malignancies at an earlier age and with a higher frequency of bilaterality than what usually occurs in the general population. Cancer is a disease of somatic cells; however, if 2 (or more) independent events are needed for the cells to become malignant, then inheriting the first step, as opposed to waiting for it to occur as a result of some environmental event or exposure causing a somatic alteration, will surely increase the likelihood of cancer occurring compared with those individuals who do not inherit such mutations. The second (and any subsequent) step is invariably somatic in nature, also explaining why not everyone who inherits a susceptibility gene (ie, mutation in a tumor suppressor gene) develops the malignancy. Molecular studies of cancers in individuals with malignancies arising from hereditary cancer syndromes frequently show a loss of heterozygosity at the genomic position of the tumor suppressor gene in tumor tissue. This loss of heterozygosity (both tumor suppressor gene copies with a mutation) is the result of the second step, and is necessary for the development of malignancies in individuals who have inherited certain cancer susceptibility gene mutations.

There are numerous mechanisms that likely lead to this loss of heterozygosity and, thus, the inactivation of the tumor suppressing gene. While cellular and nuclear somatic events are common and mostly random processes by which genes and chromosomes are altered, deleted, replaced, or rearranged without typically leading to pathology, such changes in the presence of an inherited gene mutation in a tumor suppressor gene can lead to the inactivation of tumor-suppressing gene function and predispose that organ to undergo malignant transformation. This process is known as monoallelic inheritance of a gene mutation with subsequent inactivation of the wild-type allele and loss of heterozygosity. However, it is now recognized that some individuals can inherit mutations in both alleles (either homozygous or compound heterozygous), an uncommon occurrence known as inherited biallelic mutations, which tend to present with a different clinical phenotype, including childhood cancers, than what is usually associated with monoallelic (dominant) inheritance of mutations.[51]

It is interesting that while most hereditary cancer syndromes, including HBOC syndrome, are transmitted in and present as a classic autosomal dominant inherited condition, the requirement of a second step that inactivates the remaining normal allele (biallelic inactivation) makes the cellular mechanism necessary for the promotion of carcinogenesis recessive at a cellular level, which is also observed with biallelic inheritance. However, the different phenotypes associated with biallelic inheritance compared with monoallelic inheritance bespeak a difference in the molecular biology of these 2 disease inheritance patterns, and may eventually provide valuable insight into the molecular mechanisms of cancer development.

Nonetheless, most cancers, even those associated with considerable family histories, are not associated with germline mutations. Accordingly, an alternative mechanism or mechanisms are likely responsible for the development of considerably more cases of cancer than those currently associated with germline mutations in cancer predisposition genes. Fasching and colleagues[52] propose that cancer susceptibility may be influenced by common low penetrance genetic polymorphisms, which have been associated with common disorders such as diabetes. The delineation of deleterious mutations in cancer susceptibility genes was a great leap forward in the molecular and clinical elucidation of cancer development; however, further investigations are required into the molecular processes and clinical characteristics of cancer in order to develop more effective screening, diagnostic, and therapeutic interventions that are applicable to more cancers and considerably more people than are currently affected by the identification of individuals at high risk for the development of heritable malignancies.

Assuming one has provided accurate personal and family histories, counselors can use a variety of approaches to assess risk for developing heritable cancers. Qualitative and quantitative risk assessments are how counselors determine an individual's risk for possessing a deleterious mutation in a cancer susceptibility gene and for developing cancer. Qualitative risk assessment primarily uses family and personal histories to determine an individual's risk, and incorporates a variety of personal and environmental factors including exposure to toxic substances, use of medications, pathology reports, and lifestyle issues (eg, number of pregnancies, length of time breastfeeding, and so forth) among others. An accurate qualitative assessment includes a detailed personal and family history, supported by corroborated details of the individual's personal and family history. Such details will include, but are not limited to, age of patient and family members, reproductive histories, histories of genetic disorders and major illnesses, causes of death, and lifestyle issues (eg, obesity, oral contraceptive use) that could affect morbidity and mortality as well as increasing or decreasing risk for cancer development. In addition, for family members with cancer, further detail is needed including age of diagnosis, staging and grading of tumor, and years of survival. This information should optimally be obtained from operative and pathology reports as well as medical records. All of this information can be included into

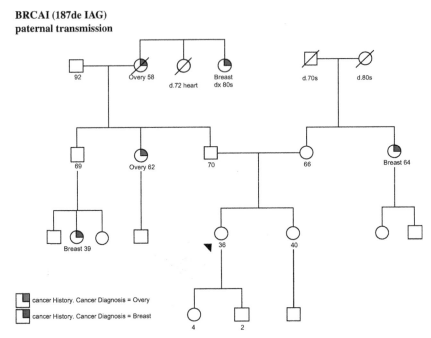

**BRCAI (187de IAG)
paternal transmission**

Fig. 3. Pedigree of individual with *BRCA1* mutation (187delAG) in proband (*arrowhead*). Transmission is through paternal side of family; father was the individual initially tested and was found to carry the deleterious mutation.

a pedigree (**Fig. 3**), which provides an easy-to-access overview of the proband and his or her family. Such information is critical even in the absence of genetic testing outcomes. Søegaard and colleagues[53] found that women with first-degree relatives with EOC were at a significantly increased risk for developing EOC, especially early-onset EOC.

Quantitative risk assessment employs risk assessment models (see section Assessing Cancer Risk) to ascertain an individual's risk for carrying a deleterious mutation in a cancer susceptibility gene. While risk assessment models are widely used to assess risk for certain cancers such as breast cancer, not all malignancies are amenable to risk assessment by a model.[54] As such, counselors usually use qualitative and quantitative approaches to determine an individual's risk for carrying a deleterious cancer susceptibility gene, and provide nondirective counseling concerning the option to undergo genetic testing or to initiate particular screening, diagnostic, or preventative measures.

In all counseling situations, counselors should also perform a psychosocial assessment of their patients, as patients frequently face emotional stress and psychological upset based on the findings of the counseling and genetic testing (if performed). Counselors should obtain information from patients before counseling and risk assessment concerning their expectations for the counseling session, the personal impact of the cancer(s) in question, and the economic impact of undergoing counseling and testing; the potential clinical outcomes, their relationship with relatives, and the ability to obtain information from those relatives; and the desire to alter their lifestyle and initiate preventative measures in case an increased risk for cancer is determined. Equally important is the sense of the patient concerning the personal and familial implications of positive or negative genetic testing results. Olaya and colleagues[55] found that 50% of individuals at increased risk for carrying a *BRCA1/2* mutation chose not to undergo genetic testing, with insurance coverage playing apparently no role in the decision to undergo or forgo such testing. In this study the investigators sought to develop counseling instruments that would better explain the benefits of testing to unaffected high-risk individuals and to target those with a high-school level education as a strategy to improve testing rates. One should consider that those individuals who chose to forgo genetic testing in this study did choose to undergo genetic counseling because of an increased risk for developing cancer. This study thus demonstrates that a variety of psychosocial factors play a major role in determining not only decisions to obtain counseling and testing but also specific choices in this informational process. Accordingly, counselors must be aware of and work with these psychosocial issues if they are to provide effective counseling and empower their patients to obtain all the information that they seek.

Testing an individual for a deleterious mutation that occurs in a parent is a relatively straightforward process; nonetheless, the emotional implications of either a positive or negative result are complex, and should be addressed before testing as the emotional impact of the testing outcomes may not necessarily be easy to predict and can profoundly impact the counseling process. A good example of this is found in the movie "In The Family" (J. Rudnick, Producer, Kartemquin Films, 2008), a film that documents the life of a *BRCA1* mutation carrier and details the lives of other individuals at risk for or with heritable breast and ovarian tumors. In one scene, 3 daughters are finding out their *BRCA1* mutation status, having decided to get tested because their mother has a deleterious *BRCA1* mutation. Two daughters are found to have inherited the mutation while the other is found to not carry the gene. Surprisingly, it is the unaffected sibling who is most upset at the findings of the genetic testing. Genetic risk assessment and testing may provide qualitative and quantitative analysis to individuals at increased risk for developing cancer; however, the perception of that risk by patients is driven by emotional and psychological factors that are considerably affected by the individual's experience with cancer. Another example of this is found in the following patient case history:

A 32-year-old woman G3P3, a college-educated, married woman with 3 children and not of Ashkenazi Jewish heritage, is referred for genetic counseling for cancer risk assessment by a Gynecologic Oncologist who saw the patient after self-referral for a bilateral salpingoophorectomy. The patient's mother had died 2 years ago from ovarian cancer at the age of 62; no other family members had ovarian cancer but several family members in the paternal and maternal families had breast cancer, with 2 paternal aunts and a first cousin with premenopausal breast cancer. After extensive counseling was provided, testing was offered to her paternal aunts with premenopausal breast cancer, who were found to carry no *BRCA1/2* mutations. Nevertheless, the patient chose to undergo *BRCA1/2* sequencing and BART (genomic rearrangement) testing, which revealed no deleterious mutations. Despite the reassuring genetic testing results, the patient was resolute in her decision to undergo extirpative ovarian surgery, even after a frank discussion of the health concerns resulting from premenopausal oophorectomy. When informed that her risk for developing breast cancer was considerably higher than her risk for developing ovarian cancer, and that bilateral mastectomy would be a risk-reducing approach to be considered, the patient look horrified and stated that she would never consider removing her breasts unless there was a malignancy.

In this situation, the patient's personal experience with her mother's ovarian cancer far outweighed her considerably higher risk for breast cancer development based on her family history. Indeed, such personal experiences are frequently the reason for certain behaviors and actions including seeking or avoiding genetic counseling, obtaining genetic testing, initiating risk-reducing interventions, and undergoing prophylactic surgeries. Many women in the Northwestern Ovarian Cancer Early Detection and Prevention Program (NOCEDPP) remain active participants in the program even after they are found not to carry the deleterious gene that was associated with a family member's (usually a parent or sibling) cancer. The discovery and acceptance of psychosocial factors in coping mechanisms, behavior modifications, and emotional reactions to medical and nonmedical events by counselors can greatly assist the counselor in providing accurate information that is best used by the patient.

The detection of a deleterious mutation provides a more clear determination of one's risk for developing cancer as well as presenting a variety of screening, diagnostic, and preventative algorithms to reduce the likelihood of cancer or to facilitate an earlier detection of cancer at a stage more amenable to successful treatment. In such cases, counselors need to be aware of the emotional implications of this finding and help their patients cope with what some describe as a personal "Sword of Damocles." Conversely, the detection of no mutation, even in individuals with parents who have mutations, can lead to unexpected emotional reactions including guilt, self-loathing, and angst, frequently as result of the concern not that they were spared but rather they were excluded from the cancer issues that beset their families. While many individuals who find they possess no deleterious mutation show positive emotions from relief to joy, assessing the psychosocial status of an individual at the beginning of the counseling process will help avert unexpected and potentially adverse reactions to risk assessment and genetic testing outcomes.

Finally, not everyone who undergoes genetic testing receives a definitive result indicating the presence or absence of a deleterious mutation. Of those undergoing testing for *BRCA1/2* mutations, approximately 7% are found to have a variant of uncertain significance (VUS). VUS are usually missense or potential splice site changes that have not, as yet, been shown to be definitively associated with adverse clinical outcomes. More than 1500 VUS have been identified, and are frequently identified in individuals of minority ethnic population. Most VUS have only been reported in 1 to 2 individuals, making further analysis of the clinical impact of VUS challenging. Once a VUS is identified, further analyses such as segregation analysis or study variants in multiple unrelated individuals are applied in an attempt to characterize the VUS as clinically relevant (favor deleterious) or irrelevant (favor polymorphism).[56] However, small sibships and family sizes as well as few individuals with any particular VUS impede the mathematical estimation needed to better characterize the clinical impact of a specific VUS.

The finding of a VUS is obviously a difficult clinical outcome that can lead to considerable emotional distress and angst concerning the clinical implications of the genetic test result. In such situations, counselors must use their skills to provide a clear and measured overview of the meaning and implication of the test, and provide emotional support for a patient who may be distraught because of the inability to obtain a definitive assessment of her risk for developing cancer.

RISK PERCEPTION AND OTHER COUNSELING ISSUES

Not surprisingly, Rantala and colleagues[57] report that prior to genetic counseling, most individuals harbor misperceptions concerning their risk, with their perception invariably being an overestimation of their actual risk. The investigators also found that there was a trend to a more accurate perception of risk following genetic counseling, and that the importance of preventative programs was well understood. According to Rantala and colleagues, cancer anxiety was prevalent and was associated with most of the inaccuracy associated with risk perception by all study participants. However, the investigators also found that cancer anxiety decreased after genetic counseling, demonstrating yet another important clinical benefit of genetic counseling for individuals at increased risk for cancer susceptibility syndromes. Similar findings were reported in an Italian study by Caruso and colleagues,[58] who also found an overestimation of cancer risk by women in this survey study compared with BRCApro calculated estimates, with more pronounced inaccuracy and misperception reported by low-risk women than high-risk women.

The anxiety observed in many people undergoing cancer genetic counseling clearly has the potential to taint the counseling process by not permitting information to be properly interpreted and analyzed by the counselee. Although this is not a unique or novel phenomenon in genetic counseling, it may be something that is not frequently encountered by medical generalists and specialists without formal genetics training. Phelps and colleagues[59] report on the development of a quantitative tool (the Genetic Risk Assessment Coping Evaluation, or GRACE) to assess the degree of distress associated with the genetic counseling risk assessment process and identify the range of coping strategies used to lessen the distress being experienced by the patient. Other tools are also available; it is important to recognize that the anxiety that leads individuals to seek counseling, and likely hinders others from initiating counseling and risk assessment, can adversely affect the counseling process if the counselor does not recognize the anxiety and does not use techniques to help individuals gain a more accurate perception of their risk and the steps to be taken, if available, to reduce their risk for developing cancer.

Morgan and colleagues[60] found that among women who had undergone genetic counseling and were at high risk for HBOC, all agreed that following cancer screening recommendations was better than not following such recommendations; none felt that the recommendations were difficult to follow and all believed that screening would help them stay healthy. More than half of the respondents (57%) believed that following the screening recommendations would prevent cancer. None reported any perceived barriers to care, although more than one-third (38%) felt that reminders would help and 10% needed assistance in following through with care. Although genetic counseling can never provide all the information needed for a decision in a manner that all patients can understand, the process of genetic counseling has clearly been shown to empower individuals to make informed decisions about critical medical issues in their lives and to provide the emotional support needed by many to follow through with their decisions.

SUMMARY

The information accrued from the Human Genome Project will surely be a revolutionary step in a process of developing new medical screening, diagnostic, and therapeutic paradigms. The delineation of the genetic and genomic characteristics of cancer, and in particular solid tumors, has altered the preventative, detection, and therapeutic approaches to these malignancies over the past decade. While much attention has been paid to the identification of tumor suppressor genes and the mutations that result in marked increases in cancer risk, there is recognition that somatic genetic alterations in tumor cells provide valuable information that is now applicable to improving clinical outcomes. For example, HER2 status in breast cancer tissue is now an important determinant in choosing the most effective chemotherapeutic regimen.[61]

This burgeoning role of genetics and genomics in the development and treatment of cancer requires professionals to be able to integrate current evidence with the ability to obtain critical information from patients and provide the necessary support to facilitate the process by which individuals at high risk are identified and offered novel screening, diagnostic, and preventative interventions to reduce the risk of cancer and improve overall clinical outcomes. Cancer genetic counseling is the process currently used to identify high-risk individuals and provide them with information and emotional support to facilitate their decision-making process. Although technological advances may eventually alter the cancer genetic counseling process, for now and the foreseeable future this will be how patients are best served in their search for answers concerning their risks for developing cancer, and in the delineation of improved interventions to prevent and treat an expanding number and variety of malignancies.

REFERENCES

1. Lancaster JM, Powell CB, Kauff ND, et al. SGO Committee Statement: Society of Gynecologic Oncologists Education Committee statement on risk assessment for inherited gynecologic cancer predispositions. Gynecol Oncol 2007;107:159–62.
2. ACOG Practice Bulletin. Hereditary breast and ovarian cancer syndrome. Gynecol Oncol 2009;113:6–11.
3. Lynch HT, Casey MJ, Snyder CL, et al. Hereditary ovarian carcinoma: heterogeneity, molecular genetics, pathology, and management. Mol Oncol 2009;3: 97–137.
4. Kjaer SK, Mellemkjaer L, Brinton LA, et al. Tubal sterilization and risk of ovarian, endometrial and cervical cancer. A Danish population-based follow-up study of more than 65,000 sterilized women. Int J Epidemiol 2004;33:596–602.
5. Palma MD, Domchek SM, Stopfer J, et al. The relative contribution of point mutations and genomic rearrangements in BRCA1 and BRCA2 in high-risk breast cancer families. Cancer Res 2008;68:7006–14.
6. Bellosillio B, Tusquets I. Pitfalls and caveats in BRCA sequencing. Ultrastruct Pathol 2006;30:229–35.
7. Whittemore AS, Gong G, Imyre J. Prevalence and contribution of BRCA1 mutations in breast cancer and ovarian cancer: results from 3 US population-based case-control studies of ovarian cancer. Am J Hum Genet 1997;60:496–504.
8. Risch HA, McLaughlin JR, Cole DEC, et al. Population BRCA1 and BRCA2 mutation frequencies and cancer penetrances: a Kin-Cohort Study in Ontario, Canada. J Natl Cancer Inst 2006;98:1694–706.
9. Metcalfe KA, Poll A, Royer R, et al. Screening for founder mutations in BRCA1 and BRCA2 in unselected Jewish women. J Clin Oncol 2010;28:387–91.
10. Mikaelsdottir EK, Valgeirsdottir S, Eyfjord JE, et al. The Icelandic founder mutation BRCA2 999del5: analysis of expression. Breast Cancer Res 2004;6:R284–90.
11. Pal T, Permuth-Wey J, Sellers TA. A review of the clinical relevance of mismatch-repair deficiency in ovarian cancer. Cancer 2008;113:733–42.
12. Wijnen J, de Leeuw W, Vasen H, et al. Familial endometrial cancer in female carriers of MSH6 germline mutations. Nat Genet 1999;23:142–4.
13. Watson P, Vasen HFA, Mecklin J-P, et al. The risk of extra-colonic, extra-endometrial cancer in the Lynch syndrome. Int J Cancer 2008;123:444–9.
14. Aaltonen LA, Peltomaki P, Leach FS, et al. Clues to the pathogenesis of familial colorectal cancer. Science 1993;260:812–6.

15. Ramus SJ, Gayther SA. The contribution of BRCA1 and BRCA2 to ovarian cancer. Mol Oncol 2009;3:138–50.

16. Bewtra C, Watson P, Conway T, et al. Hereditary ovarian cancer: a clinicopathological study. Int J Gynecol Pathol 1992;11:180–7.

17. Antoniou AC, Gayther SA, Stratton JF, et al. Risk models for familial ovarian and breast cancer. Genet Epidemiol 2000;18:173–90.

18. Brose MS, Rebbeck TR, Calzone KA, et al. Cancer risk estimates for BRCA1 mutation carriers. J Natl Cancer Inst 2002;94:1365–72.

19. The Breast Cancer Linkage Consortium. Cancer risks in BRCA2 mutation carriers. J Natl Cancer Inst 1999;91(15):1310–6.

20. Risch HA, McLaughlin JR, Cole DEC, et al. Prevalence and penetrance in germline BRCA1 and BRCA2 mutations in a population series of 649 women with ovarian cancer. Am J Hum Genet 2001;68:700–10.

21. Satagopan JM, Boyd J, Kauff ND, et al. Ovarian cancer risk in Ashkenazi Jewish carriers of BRCA1 and BRCA2 mutations. Clin Cancer Res 2002;8:3776–81.

22. Levy-Lahad E, Friedman E. Cancer risks among BRCA1 and BRCA2 mutation carriers. Br J Cancer 2007;96:11–5.

23. Mohammad HB, Apffelstaedt JP. Counseling for male BRCA mutation carriers— a review. Breast 2008;17:441–50.

24. Ostrander EA, Udler MS. The role of the BRCA2 gene in susceptibility to prostate cancer revisited. Cancer Epidemiol Biomarkers Prev 2008;17:1843–8.

25. Brose M, Rebbeck T, Calzone K, et al. Cancer risk estimates for BRCA1 mutation carriers identified in a cancer risk evaluation program. J Natl Cancer Inst 2002;94:1359–65.

26. Mai PL, Chatterjee N, Hartge P, et al. Potential excess mortality in BRCA1/2 mutation carriers beyond breast, ovarian, prostate and pancreatic cancers, and melanoma. PLoS One 2009;4(3):e4812. DOI: 10.1371/journal.pone.0004812.

27. Lynch HT, Lynch PM, Lanspa SJ, et al. Review of the Lynch syndrome: history, molecular genetics, screening, differential diagnosis, and medicolegal ramifications. Clin Genet 2009;76:1–18.

28. Aarnio M, Sankila R, Pukkala E, et al. Cancer risk in mutation carriers of DNA mismatch repair genes. Int J Cancer 1999;81:214–8.

29. Banno K, Yanokura M, Kobayashi Y, et al. Endometrial cancer as a familial tumor: pathology and molecular carcinogenesis [review]. Curr Genomics 2009;10:127–32.

30. Mathews KS, Estes JM, Connor MG, et al. Lynch syndrome in women less than 50 years of age with endometrial cancer. Obstet Gynecol 2008;111:1161–6.

31. Malander S, Rambech E, Kristoffersson U, et al. The contribution of the hereditary nonpolyposis colorectal cancer syndrome to the development of ovarian cancer. Gynecol Oncol 2006;101:238–43.

32. Russo A, Calo V, Bruno L, et al. Hereditary ovarian cancer. Crit Rev Oncol Hematol 2009;69:28–44.

33. Cederquist K, Emanuelsson M, Wiklund F, et al. Two Swedish founder MSH6 mutations, one nonsense and one missense, conferring high cumulative risk of Lynch syndrome. Clin Genet 2005;68:533–41.

34. Hampel H, Frankel WL, Martin E, et al. Feasibility of screening for Lynch syndrome among patients with colorectal cancer. J Clin Oncol 2008;26:5783–8.

35. Jordan SK, Siskind V, Green C, et al. Breastfeeding and risk of epithelial ovarian cancer. Cancer Causes Control 2010;21:109–16.

36. Kurian AW, Sigal BM, Plevritis SK. Survival analysis of cancer risk reduction strategies for BRCA1/2 mutation carriers. J Clin Oncol 2010;28:222–31.

37. U.S. Preventive Services Task Force. Genetic risk assessment and BRCA mutation testing for breast and ovarian cancer susceptibility: recommendation statement. Ann Intern Med 2005;143:355–61.

38. Santen RJ, Boyd NF, Chlebowski RT, et al. Critical assessment of new risk factors for breast cancer: considerations for development of an improved risk prediction model. Endocr Relat Cancer 2007;14:169–87.

39. South SA, Vance H, Farrell C, et al. Consideration of hereditary nonpolyposis colorectal cancer in BRCA mutation-negative familial ovarian cancers. Cancer 2009;115:324–33.

40. Vasen HF, Hendriks Y, de Jong AE, et al. Identification of HNPCC by molecular analysis of colon and endometrial tumors. Dis Markers 2004;20:207–13.

41. Resnick KE, Hampel H, Fishel R, et al. Current and emerging trends in Lynch syndrome identification in women with endometrial cancer. Gynecol Oncol 2009;114:128–34.

42. Goodfellow PJ, Buttin BM, Herzog TJ, et al. Prevalence of defective DNA mismatch repair and MSH6 mutation in an unselected series of endometrial cancers. Proc Natl Acad Sci U S A 2003;100:5908–13.

43. Hampel H, Panescu J, Lockman J, et al. Comment on: screening for Lynch syndrome (hereditary nonpolyposis colon cancer) among endometrial cancer patients. Cancer Res 2007;62:9603.

44. Allain DC. Genetic counseling and testing for common hereditary breast cancer syndromes. J Mol Diagn 2008;10:383–95.

45. Orloff MS, Eng C. Genetic and phenotypic heterogeneity in the PTEN hamartoma tumour syndrome. Oncogene 2008;27:5387–97.

46. Eng C. Will the real Cowden syndrome please stand up: revised diagnostic criteria. J Med Genet 2000;37:828–30.

47. Shulman LP. Advances in female hormonal contraception: current alternatives to oral regimens. Treat Endocrinol 2003;2:247–56.

48. Lustbader ED, Williams WR, Bondy ML, et al. Segregation analysis of cancer in families of childhood soft-tissue-sarcoma patients. Am J Hum Genet 1992;51:344–56.

49. Kinsler KW, Vogelstein B. Lessons from hereditary colorectal cancer. Cell 1996;87:159–70.

50. Knudson AG. Two genetic hits (more or less) to cancer. Nat Rev Cancer 2001;1:157–62.

51. Rahman N, Scott RH. Cancer genes associated with phenotypes in monoallelic and biallelic mutation carriers: new lessons from old players. Hum Mol Genet 2007;16(Spec No 1):R60–6.

52. Fasching PA, Gayther S, Pearce L, et al. Role of genetic polymorphisms and ovarian cancer susceptibility. Mol Oncol 2009;3:171–81.

53. Søegaard M, Frederiksen K, Jensen A, et al. Risk of ovarian cancer in women with first-degree relatives with cancer. Acta Obstet Gynecol Scand 2009;88:449–56.

54. Prucka SK, McIlvried DE, Korf BR. Cancer risk assessment and the genetic counseling process: using hereditary breast and ovarian cancer as an example. Med Princ Pract 2008;17:173–89.

55. Olaya W, Esquivel P, Wong JH, et al. Disparities in BRCA testing: when insurance coverage is not a barrier. Am J Surg 2009;198:562–5.

56. Spearman AD, Sweet K, Zhou X-P, et al. Clinically applicable models to characterize BRCA1 and BRCA2 variants of uncertain significance. J Clin Oncol 2008;26:5393–400.

57. Rantala J, Platten U, Lindgren G, et al. Risk perception after genetic counseling in patients with increased risk of cancer. Hered Cancer Clin Pract 2009;7:15.
58. Caruso A, Vigna C, Marozzo B, et al. Subjective versus objective risk in genetic counseling for hereditary breast and/or ovarian cancers. J Exp Clin Cancer Res 2009;28:157.
59. Phelps C, Bennett P, Jones H, et al. The development of a cancer genetic-specific measure of coping: the GRACE. Psychooncology 2009. DOI: 10.1002/pon.1629.
60. Morgan D, Sylvester H, Lucas FL, et al. Perceptions of high-risk care and barriers to care among women at risk for hereditary breast and ovarian cancer following genetic counseling in the community setting. J Genet Couns 2009. DOI: 10.1007/s10897-009-9261-9.
61. Osako T, Horii R, Matsuura M, et al. High-grade breast cancers include both highly sensitive and highly resistant subsets to cytotoxic chemotherapy. J Cancer Res Clin Oncol 2010 Feb 9. [Epub ahead of print].

Erratum

An error appeared in the article "Pharmacologic Management of Urinary Incontinence, Voiding Dysfunction, and Overactive Bladder" in the September 2009 issue of *Obstetrics and Gynecology Clinics of North America* (Volume 36, Issue 3). **Fig. 1** in the original article should be replaced with the figure below:

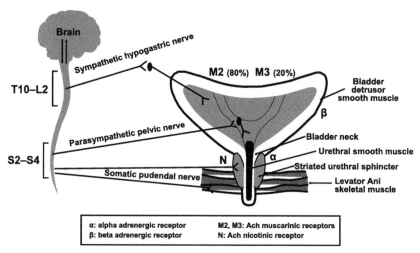

Fig. 1. Neurophysiology of the lower urinary tract. *Adapted from* Wein AJ. Pharmacological agents for the treatment of urinary incontinence due to overactive bladder. Expert Opin Investig Drugs 2001;10(1):65–83; with permission. *Data from* Abrams P, Andersson KE, Buccafusco JJ, et al. Muscarinic receptors: their distribution and function in body systems, and the implications for treating overactive bladder. Br J Pharmacol 2006;148(5):565–78; and Benson JT, Walters MD. Neurophysiology and pharmacology of the lower urinary tract. In: Walters MD, Karram MM, editors. Urogynecology and Reconstructive Surgery. 3rd edition. Philadelphia: Elsevier; 2007. p. 33.

Obstet Gynecol Clin N Am 37 (2010) 135
doi:10.1016/j.ogc.2010.04.023
0889-8545/10/$ – see front matter © 2010 Elsevier Inc. All rights reserved.

obgyn.theclinics.com

Index

Note: Page numbers of article titles are in **boldface** type.

A

aCGH. See *Array comparative genomic hybridization (aCGH).*
Adrenal hyperplasia, congenital, NBS for, 18
Allele(s), fragile X. See *Fragile X allele; Fragile X allele carriers.*
Amino acid disorders, NBS for, 16
Ancestry-based carrier screening, 4–5
Anticoagulant(s), natural, in thrombophilia, 94–95
Antithrombin III, in thrombophilia, 94
Array comparative genomic hybridization (aCGH)
    benefits of, 77
    clinical diagnostic use of, 77
    in genetic counseling, 81–82
    in genomic disorders, discovery and delineation uses, 75–77
    in obstetrics, **71–85**
    in pregnancy loss, cytogenetic analysis, 80–81
    limitations of, 77–78
    prenatal experience with, successes/limitations, 78–80
    principles of, 73–74
    single nucleotide polymorphism arrays, basis of, 75
Ashkenazi Jewish screening. See also *Jewish populations.*
    in twenty-first century, **37–46**
        current recommendations, 43–44
Assisted reproduction, contemporary genetic counseling for, 6–7

B

Biology, HBOC–related, 110–113
Biotinidase deficiency, NBS for, 18
Bloom syndrome, in Jewish populations, 41, 43
BRCA1, biology of, 110–112
BRCA2, biology of, 110–112
Breast cancer, hereditary cancer syndromes associated with, 121–123

C

Canavan disease, in Jewish populations, 40–42
Cancer(s). See specific types.
Carrier screening
    ancestry-based, 4–5
    for cystic fibrosis, **47–59**. See also *Cystic fibrosis, carrier screening for.*

Obstet Gynecol Clin N Am 37 (2010) 137–142
doi:10.1016/S0889-8545(10)00038-0
0889-8545/10/$ – see front matter © 2010 Elsevier Inc. All rights reserved.

obgyn.theclinics.com

Moving?

Make sure your subscription moves with you!

To notify us of your new address, find your **Clinics Account Number** (located on your mailing label above your name), and contact customer service at:

Email: **journalscustomerservice-usa@elsevier.com**

800-654-2452 (subscribers in the U.S. & Canada)
314-447-8871 (subscribers outside of the U.S. & Canada)

Fax number: 314-447-8029

Elsevier Health Sciences Division
Subscription Customer Service
3251 Riverport Lane
Maryland Heights, MO 63043

*To ensure uninterrupted delivery of your subscription, please notify us at least 4 weeks in advance of move.